The Atkins Diet Weight Loss Solution

Essential Beginner's Guidebook with Kickstart Meal Plan and Low Carb Recipes Full of Healthy Fats

Adele Baker

Copyright © 2019 by Adele Baker.

All rights reserved.

No part of this book may be reproduced in any form or by any electronic or mechanical means, except in the case of a brief quotation embodied in articles or reviews, without written permission from its publisher.

Disclaimer

The recipes and information in this book are provided for educational purposes only. Please always consult a licensed professional before making changes to your lifestyle or diet. The author and publisher shall have neither liability nor responsibility to anyone with respect to any loss or damage caused or alleged to be caused directly or indirectly by the information contained in this book. All trademarks and brands within this book are for clarifying purposes only and are owned by the owners themselves, not affiliated with this document.

Images from shutterstock.com

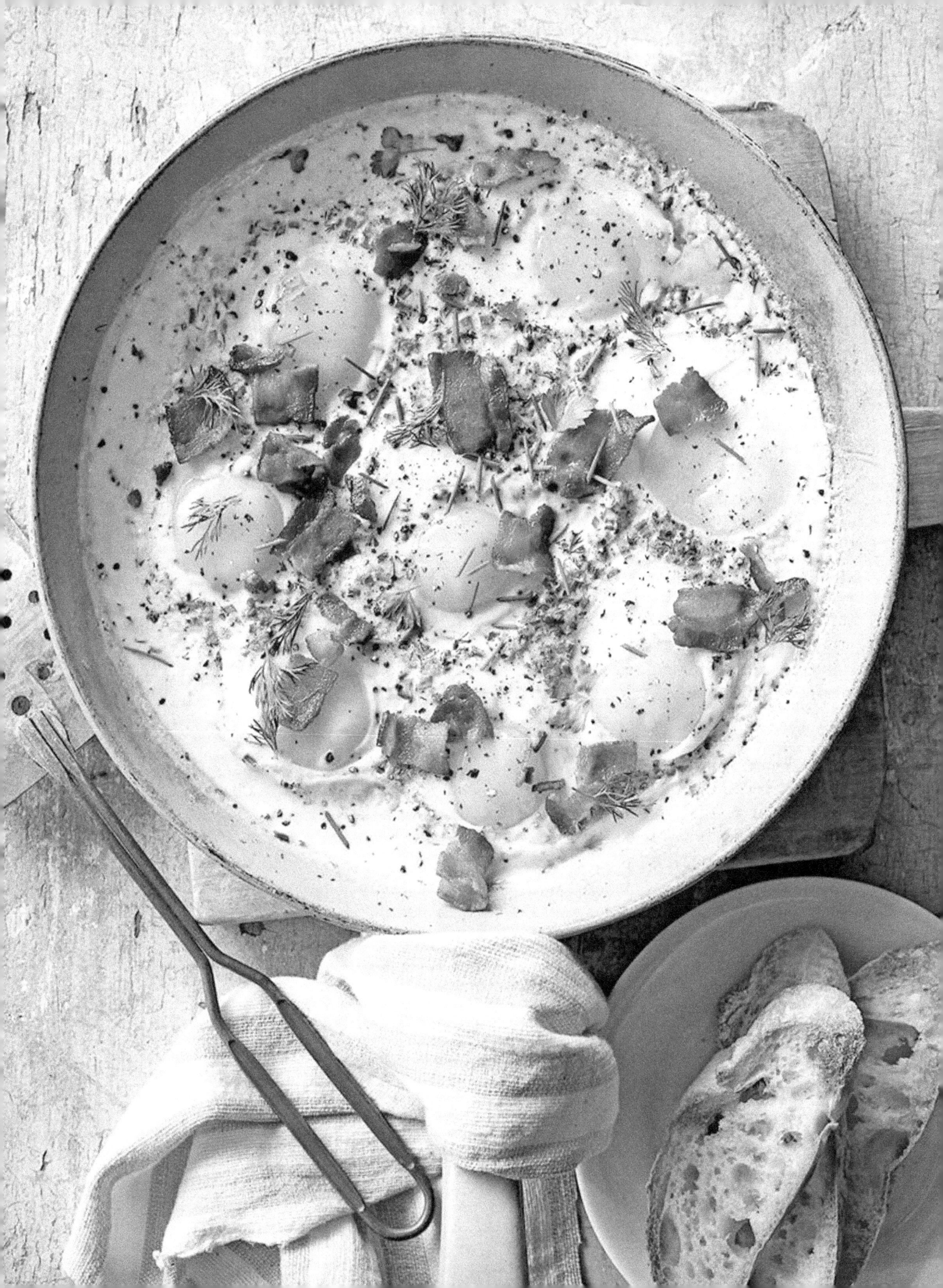

CONTENTS

INTRODUCTION 6

Chapter 1. The Basics 7
    What is the New Atkins Diet 7
    Foods to Eat and Avoid 8
    Pros and Cons of the Atkins Diet 9
    Myths and Facts about the New Atkins Diet 13
    Smart Shopping Strategies 14

Chapter 2. Three-Week Atkins Meal Plan 16

Chapter 3. Recipes 19

BREAKFAST 19
    Belgian Waffles 19
    Flaxseed Pancake 20
    Whole-Wheat Currant Scones 21
    Peanut-Strawberry Breakfast Bars 22
    Crunchy Tropical Berry and Almond Breakfast Parfait 23
    Cauliflower Rice Scrambles 24
    Broiler Huevos Rancheros 25
    Cheese Pancake 26
    Cranberry-Orange Loaf 27
    Pancakes With Ricotta-Apricot Filling 28
    Atkins Yorkshire Pudding 29
    Birdies in a Basket 30

VEGETABLES AND OTHER SIDES 31
    Sautéed Greens with Pecans 31
    Stir-Fried Broccolini with Cashews 32
    Roasted Lemon-Garlic Brussels Sprouts 33
    Sautéed Baby Bok Choy with Garlic and Lemon Zest 34
    Swiss Chard with Pine Nuts 35
    Braised Lettuce 36
    Roasted Cauliflower 37
    Sautéed Spinach with Caramelized Shallots 38
    Shishito Peppers with Hot Paprika Mayonnaise 39
    Asparagus with Burrata Cheese and Kale Pesto 40

SOUPS AND STEWS 41
    Jalapeño Cheddar Broccoli Soup 41
    Cauliflower Bisque 42
    Spicy Korean Soup with Scallions 43
    Salsa Verde Chicken Soup 44
    Chicken Vegetable Soup 45
    Thai Coconut-Shrimp Soup 46
    Chinese Hot-and-Sour Soup 47
    Creamy Cheddar Cheese Soup 48

Cream of Broccoli Soup...49
Cold Roasted Tomato Soup...50

SALADS 51

Athenian Salad 51
Caprese Salad 52
Old Bay Shrimp Salad 53
Watercress Bacon Salad with Ranch Dressing 54
Shaved Fennel Salad with Lemon Dressing 55
Cucumber-Dill Salad..56
Slaw with Vinegar Dressing 57
Wedge Salad with Gorgonzola Dressing 58
Mixed Power Greens Prosciutto-Wrapped Chicken Tenders 59
Tomato and Red Onion Salad 60

MAIN DISHES 61

Mushroom-Herb-Stuffed Chicken Breasts 61
Jerk Chicken..62
Roast Beef with Greek Yogurt- Horseradish Sauce 63
Chicken-Fried Steak 64
Slow-Cooked Pork Shoulder 65
Fontina-and-Prosciutto-Stuffed Veal Chops 66
Almond-Crusted Catfish Fingers 67
Baked Bluefish with Garlic and Lime 68
Baked Salmon with Mustard-Nut Crust 69
Beef Bourguignon..70
Roasted Fennel and Cod with Moroccan Olives...71
Year-Round Barbecued Brisket 72
Salmon with Rosemary 73

DESSERTS 74

Chocolate Chip Cookies..74
Chocolate-Orange Soufflés...75
Lickety-Split Vanilla Ice Cream 76
Cranberry-Orange Fool 77
Mini-Muffin-Tin Chocolate Brownies...78
Vanilla Meringues 79
Apple Crumble 80
Double Chocolate Brownies 81
Salted Caramel Cheesecake Bites 82
Mexican Wedding Cookies 83

CONCLUSION 84

Recipe Index 85

Conversion Tables 86

Other Books by Adele Baker 87

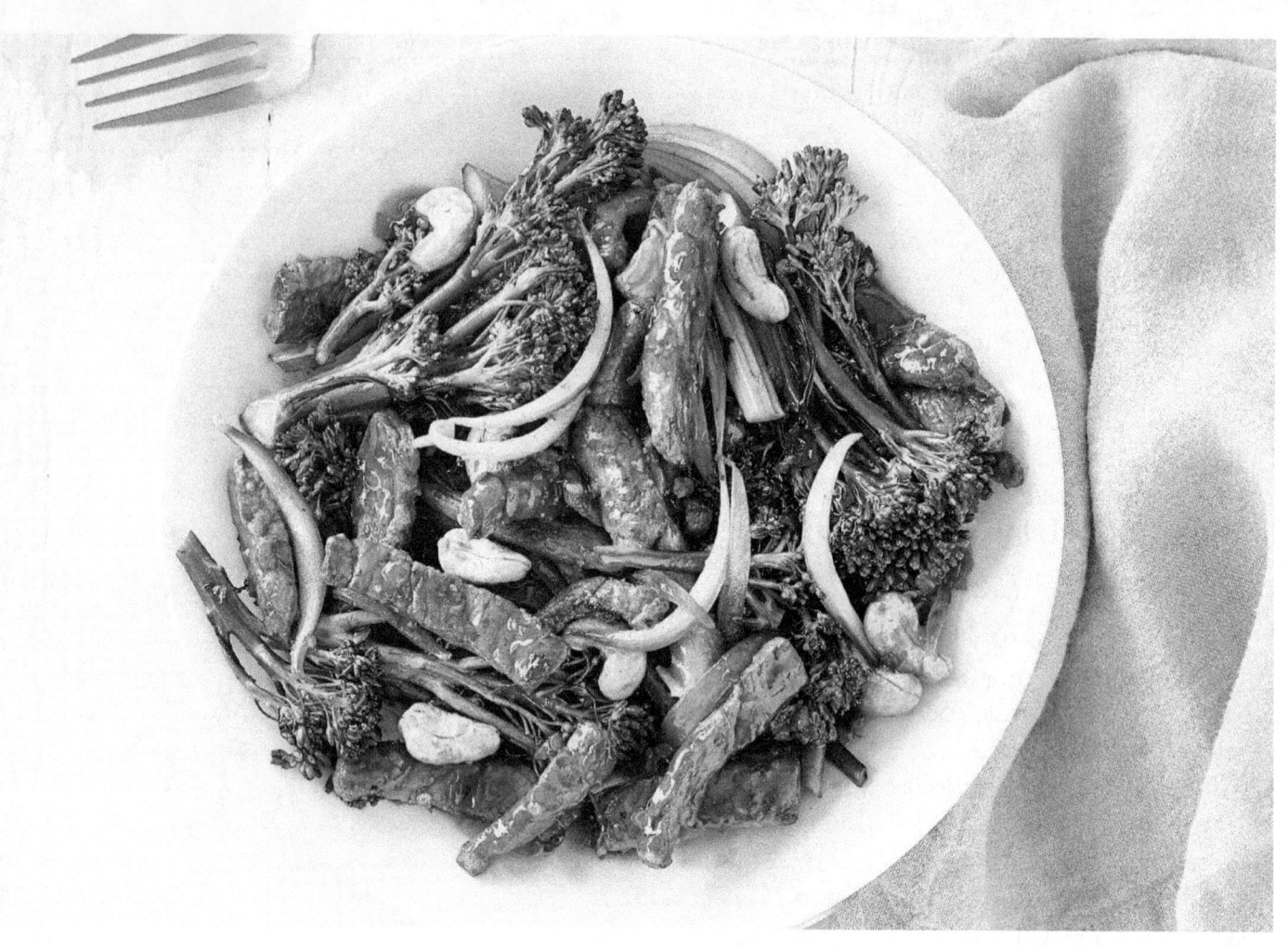

INTRODUCTION

Lose weight! Increase energy! Look great! This book will help you with all this. It will show you how to change your life once and for all. The New Atkins Diet is the program you've been looking for.

The New Atkins Diet is different from the typical American way of eating. It offers a better, smarter way to help you become healthier and fit. Being on Atkins, you avoid the negative consequences of too much carbohydrate intake, which is connected with too much insulin release in your body. In the last few years, more than fifty studies have shown new insights into ways to optimize the Atkins lifestyle, validating the safety and effectiveness of this nutritional program.

This book contains proven steps and strategies on how to use the Atkins diet program to achieve your desired weight and be in the best possible shape. While reading this book, you will figure out what diet mistakes you may have been committing and how you can change things, understand what the New Atkins Diet is all about, get to know each phase of the Atkins diet and ways to maximize your weight loss results every step of the way. On top of it all, you will get a three-week meal plan that can make you lose weight while enjoying delicious meals and a lot of tasty and easy recipes to make.

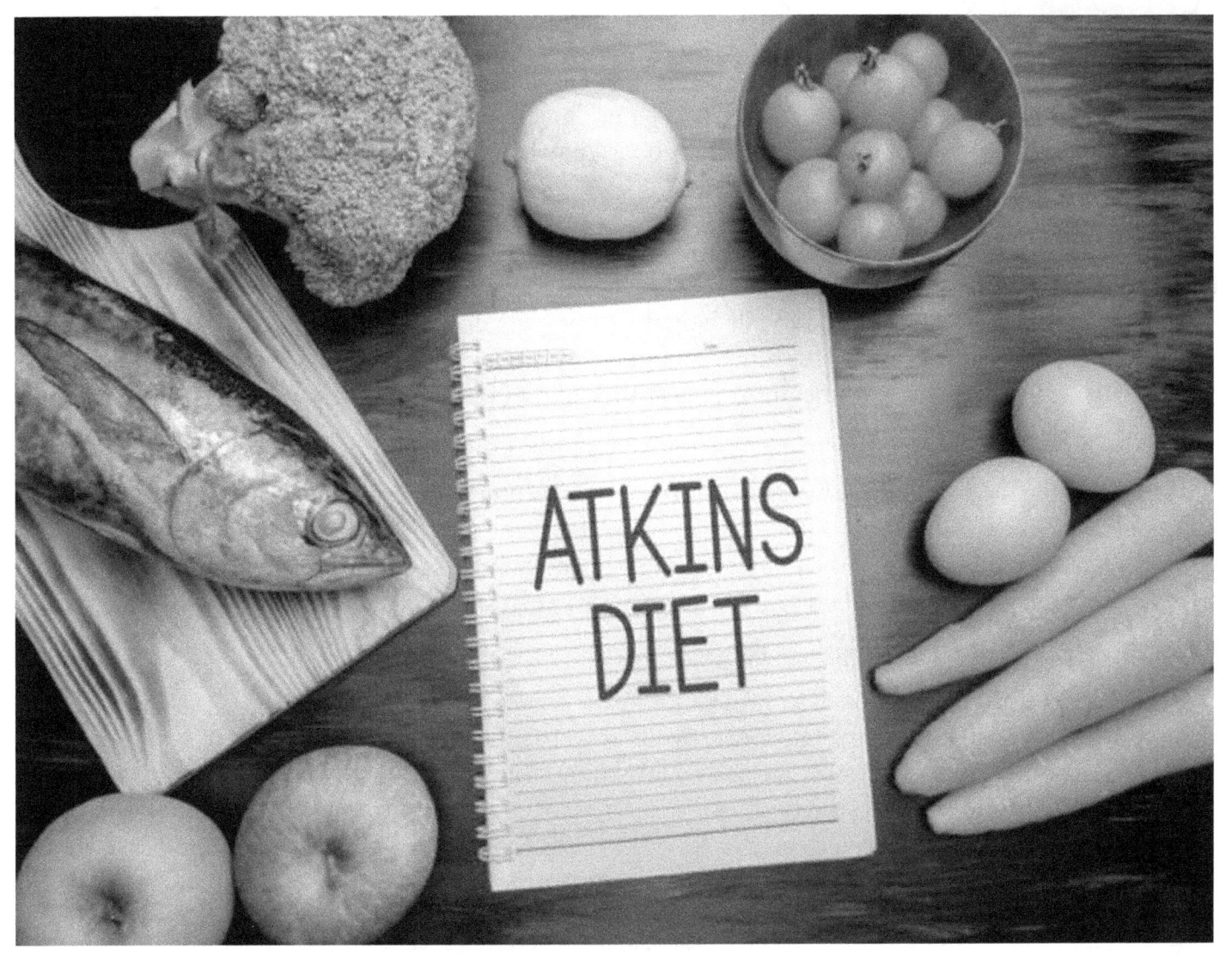

Chapter 1. The Basics

What is the New Atkins Diet

The Atkins diet is the most successful weight loss and weight maintenance program of the last quarter of the twentieth century. The Atkins diet started its development when cardiologist Dr. Robert Atkins refuted conventional wisdom that claimed losing weight is only possible by cutting calories and fat. Such eating principles turned into a vicious cycle that left us feeling deprived and then overeating. Dr. Atkins discovered that when you take slow but confident steps to cut back on carbohydrates (carbs) and sugar, you transform your metabolism from one that stores fat into one that burns fat. For years, we've been assured that fat is the main reason for the obesity epidemic. We ate low-fat cookies and drank skim milk. But we still were getting fatter. But fat is not the enemy. There is another reason that lurks in many of the "healthful" foods we eat and drink. And guess what: it's sugar and excess carbohydrates.

The New Atkins Diet represents principles that Dr. Robert C. Atkins set forth four decades ago but includes changes for greater flexibility. Some of these subtle but substantial shifts are simply the result of a greater understanding of human metabolism and food science.The Atkins diet can have a positive effect on the lives of people facing the risk factors associated with heart disease, diabetes, and hypertension.

There are a few key points you need to understand in order to put Atkins into action correctly.

You don't need to count calories on Atkins.

The quality and quantity of the protein, fats, and carbohydrates that you eat while on Atkins are most important. The only thing you count on Atkins is your daily grams of Net Carbs, which helps ensure that you are eating the high-quality, nutrient-rich foods that keep you full and satisfied, so your calories naturally fall into a healthy range.

Atkins is not a high-protein plan.

Though you'll be eating adequate amounts of protein, Atkins' typical intake of about 65 to 175 grams (2-6 oz) of protein a day, depending on your height, is not considered high protein. Think of Atkins as a nutritional approach that features "optimal" amounts of protein. Your ideal amount of protein will make you feel full after your meal, not uncomfortably stuffed and not hungry until your next scheduled meal.

Atkins has built-in portion control.

You will be eating foods that contain necessary amounts of protein, good fat and fiber, helping you achieve your goals while controlling your hunger. This is because these foods are naturally self-limiting. Almost everyone has probably scarfed down half a package of cookies or a bag of chips in one sitting, but have you ever overdone it on hard-boiled eggs or steamed broccoli?

Let's headline the general principles of the New Atkins Diet:

- ✓ Atkins is a lifetime approach to eating, not just a weight loss diet
- ✓ Curb your carb intake, and you convert your body to burning primarily fat for energy
- ✓ When you begin to tap into your body's fat stores, you thwart the metabolic bully that normally blocks access to your fat stores
- ✓ This metabolic adaptation, known as the Atkins Edge, provides a steady source of energy, helping control your appetite and eliminating or reducing carb cravings
- ✓ You'll lose water weight first on Atkins, as you do on any weight loss diet, but fat loss will quickly follow
- ✓ Consuming a modest amount of salt eliminates or moderates symptoms that may accompany the diet's diuretic effect and the metabolic shift to burning fat
- ✓ The amount and quality of the carbohydrate foods you eat impact the amount of insulin in your bloodstream
- ✓ Fat is easily stored in your body, but there is limited storage space for carbohydrate, so any excess converts to fat

Foods to Eat and Avoid

List of foods to eat:

- Pastured eggs mostly from chicken and turkey among others
- Full-fat dairy products
- Meats such as beef, bacon, and pork
- Vegetables low in carbs, including asparagus, kale, broccoli, cauliflower, green beans, cabbage, Brussels sprouts, canned cucumber, zucchini, lettuce, bell peppers and jalapeño peppers.
- Seafood and fatty fish. Wild-caught fish is recommended. Avoid shellfish, including shrimp. The best choices are haddock, trout and salmon.
- Avocados
- Seeds and nuts

- Healthy fats like virgin coconut and avocado oils
- Herbs and spices such as cayenne pepper, curry powder, thyme, cumin, paprika, cinnamon, five spice powder, oregano, chili powder, Dijon mustard, basil, parsley, tarragon, garlic (both whole and ground) and black pepper.
- Hard cheese, both sour and heavy cream (it is recommended you choose the grass-fed as well as organic if possible, which is made from raw milk), and butter. When it comes to cheese products the most approved ones are goat, cheddar, parmesan, blue cheese, Swiss and feta.
- When it comes to drinks, it is recommended to opt for water, green tea, and coffee

Dieters are advised to avoid the following foods:
- Sugar, as well as anything composed of artificial sweeteners or added sweeteners such as those found in cakes, soft drinks and candy
- Legumes like lentils, chickpeas, and beans
- Grains such as rice, wheat or any other whole grains. While on this diet, also avoid any food that is made with grain flour, including biscuits, cereal, bread, cakes, muffin, pasta and much more.
- Low-fat foods because they may have high sugar levels
- Some premade condiments such as sauces or packet mixes since they tend to have high sugar levels.
- Most fruits as well as fruit juices. It is okay though to have limes or lemons
- All foods which have been made with hydrogenated oils. This kind of food includes most of the junk foods or famously known as fast/fried foods.
- Diet foods which have artificial ingredients and reduced fat. These products have some extra thickener, sweetener or carbs to make up for the lost fat.
- Some dairy products which contain milk, cottage cheese, yogurt or ricotta. You are allowed to have higher-fat and low-carb cheeses as they contain minimal carbs.
- Starchy veggies including carrots, butternut/winter squash, potatoes and parsnips

Pros and Cons of the Atkins Diet

The Atkins diet may cause weight loss, but some people still ask if the diet is necessarily healthy? All diets tend to have different effects on various kinds of people, for example, on women and men. It most likely will not be a good fit for every person, but most of the diets which are low in carbs have some health benefits. Let us first look at the health benefits of being on the New Atkins Diet:

1. **Low-carb diet helps to curb your appetite**

One common and bad side effect of being on a diet is the feeling of hunger. It is one of the reasons which cause individuals to feel miserable when on their diets causing them to eventually give it up. Eating a low-carb diet naturally reduces your appetite and cravings for all those foods that you might have thought you cannot live without. So how does it work?

There is an effect on your blood insulin levels each time you eat a low-carb meal. The levels will drop dramatically, which in turn will lead to the suppressing effect on your appetite. Eating carbs will have the opposite effect. It will result in spikes in your insulin levels which then will lead to massive cravings and heightened appetite. You know how bad it can be when you crave and eat more unhealthy foods. Aside from just gaining weight, it can also lead to very critical health issues— diabetes being one of them.

Seeing the world today with so many people seeking to keep their weight in check, there is a high demand for chemical appetite suppressants as well as the natural ones. But does it make sense for someone to take something out of a bottle when they can simply eat properly? It is very rare to hear someone who is on a low-carb diet "being hungry." Therefore when you cut carbs, your appetite will decrease, and you will consume much fewer calories even without putting in an effort.

2. A greater proportion of the fat you lose will come from your abdominal cavity

Abdominal fat has been linked to a higher risk of heart disease. Not all the fat in your body is the same. Where the fat is stored is what will determine to what extent it will affect your health and put you at risk of certain diseases. We all have two types of fat, the subcutaneous fat which is found under the skin and the visceral fat which is found in the abdominal cavity. When it comes to visceral fat, it tends to settle around your organs, and this is not a good thing. When you have a lot of fat in that particular area, it can result in inflammation and insulin resistance. When on a diet over time, you will be able to reduce drastically your risk of heart disease as well as type 2 diabetes.

Research has also proven it to be one of the leading causes of metabolic dysfunction which is becoming very common in the developed countries of the world today. One of the proven and very effective ways that you can reduce your abdominal fat is with low-carb diets such as the Atkins diet. These diets are even responsible for more fat loss than the low-fat diets. Furthermore, the low-carb diet targets a greater proportion of the fat in the abdominal cavity.

3. It leads to more weight loss

I do not see any other way which is as simple and as efficient in helping you to lose weight than cutting down on carbs. Studies have also been able to confirm this fact, showing that individuals who are on a low-carb diet lose more weight at a much faster rate when compared to those on a low-fat diet. The low-carb diet still prevails even when those on a low-fat diet are also actively restricting their calories.

One reason is that a low-carb diet tends to make you get rid of the excess water in your body. As a result, it will lead to lowering the insulin levels which cause the kidneys to start shedding the excess sodium. As seen earlier, it is because of this reason that a person will lose weight fast during the first couple of weeks on the diet. Some studies have also compared the low-carb with the low-fat diets; the result is that those dieters who are on a low-carb diet will lose twice or thrice the weight those on the low-fat diet lose and without feeling hungry. It is without a doubt that the low-carb diets will help you to lose more weight than the other diets, especially in your first six months.

4. It reduces your blood pressure

Having high blood pressure levels, or hypertension, is one of the important risk factors for some diseases. Well, one way you can help reduce your blood pressure might just be by going on a low-carb diet. It is an efficient method which will lead to a reduced risk of some common diseases. Researchers say that just losing weight by itself will typically lead to a real reduction in your blood pressure. But it appears that a diet which is low in carbohydrates also has an additional effect on helping to lower blood pressure.

According to research experts, the weight and shape of your body will affect your blood pressure and also the risk of developing strokes and heart disease. The general rule here is that the greater your body weight is above normal, the higher the chances of having higher blood pressure. The first thing that anyone who has high blood pressure is advised to do is to try and maintain a healthy body weight. Often it is the abdominal fat that is responsible for causing the problem. Using a low-carbohydrate diet such as the Atkins diet, may work better than "fat-removal pills" when it comes to lowering your blood pressure.

5. The diet improves the LDL-cholesterol pattern

The Low-Density Lipoprotein is a protein which is also known as the "bad" cholesterol. Those individuals who have a high LDL are more likely to have heart attacks. Specialists have pointed out that the actual number of LDL is not all that helpful when it comes to predicting who will go on to have heart disease. The discovery of the LDL particle size pattern has made it possible for physicians to have more information about how bad the LDL of an individual is.

When the LDL particles are small, it makes it easier to predict coronary artery disease than when the particles are large. The particle size pattern usually improves when a person is on a low-carb diet. In studies where people were switched to a low-carb diet, the patterns changed in a favorable direction. It reduces the number of LDL particles that are floating around in your bloodstream.

6. The most effective treatment against Metabolic Syndrome

If you are not familiar with the Metabolic Syndrome, it consists of symptoms which put you at risk for heart disease. It consists of some metabolic risk factors which will appear together. Over quite some time now, many people have been turning to the Atkins dietary strategy of reduced sugar and carbohydrates because of its ability to help individuals lose weight and keep it off as well. But the Atkins diet can accomplish even more than just that as shown by on-going research over and over again.

The findings are that the diet can lower an inflammation marker, improve cholesterol ratios, and improve both insulin sensitivity and the control of blood glucose as well as a dramatic improvement of triglyceride readings. Now the studies also show that the Atkins diet is effective for improving measures of the metabolic syndrome, a severe condition. A low-carb diet will provide you with a greater overall improvement of Metabolic Syndrome risk factors than the low-fat diet with reduced calorie intake.

7. Reduces the risk of Dementia

One of the ways to fight cognitive problems such as dementia, narcolepsy and Alzheimer's disease is with a low-carb diet. Studies show that individuals who experience a higher resistance to insulin have a greater chance of demonstrating inflammation and significantly lower circulation of blood to the brain and, as a result, a lower brain plasticity or adaptability

Dangers and Precautions Related With the Atkins Diet

As a beginner of the diet, do you have to be concerned with the risks, if any, that it might cause,? And if there are any, what are the various precautions that you should take? One of the biggest flaws of the Atkins diet is that it mostly cuts out both the healthy and unhealthy carbs and replaces them with cheese, poultry, and high-fat meats.

Although dieters who are on Atkins receive results, there is no single approach to low-carb dieting that will work correctly for all people to improve their health as well as quality of life. Losing weight is not all there is when one goes on a diet; the diet should also be sustainable as well as something that will benefit your mind and body. If you feel too restricted by your diet, then the chances are greater that you are going to gain more weight than you lost with the diet.

There are many factors which can cause you to find the Atkins diet to be difficult to follow or to be rewarding. These factors include your age, medical history, your level of activity, gender, genetic disposition, and body weight. Some studies show that the diet plan can lead to stomach problems or cause cognitive symptoms when compared to dieters who are on a low-fat diet plan. There are possibilities of side effects when on a low-carb diet. You need to know that the possible side effects do not occur with everybody and their severity can also vary from one person to the next. The effects are such as:

- Bad breath
- Indigestion which is caused by eating too much fat
- Having trouble sleeping

- Mood swings or feeling irritated which can happen when a person reduces their carb intake which can affect serotonin levels
- Fatigue
- Digestive problems such as constipation caused by low intake of fiber
- Difficulties exercising as a result of feeling weak or losing interest in being active because of feeling tired

Just like any other dietary plan, it is most important that you learn to be self-aware, especially if you intend to reduce the carb intake drastically to lose weight. This is particularly true for those individuals who are old, very physically active those who have a hormone-related health problem, are underweight, pregnant or breastfeeding. To get the level of carbs in your diet which works best for you, you should pay much attention to your sleep, how you feel, energy, digestion, and moods as we will see in the next chapter.

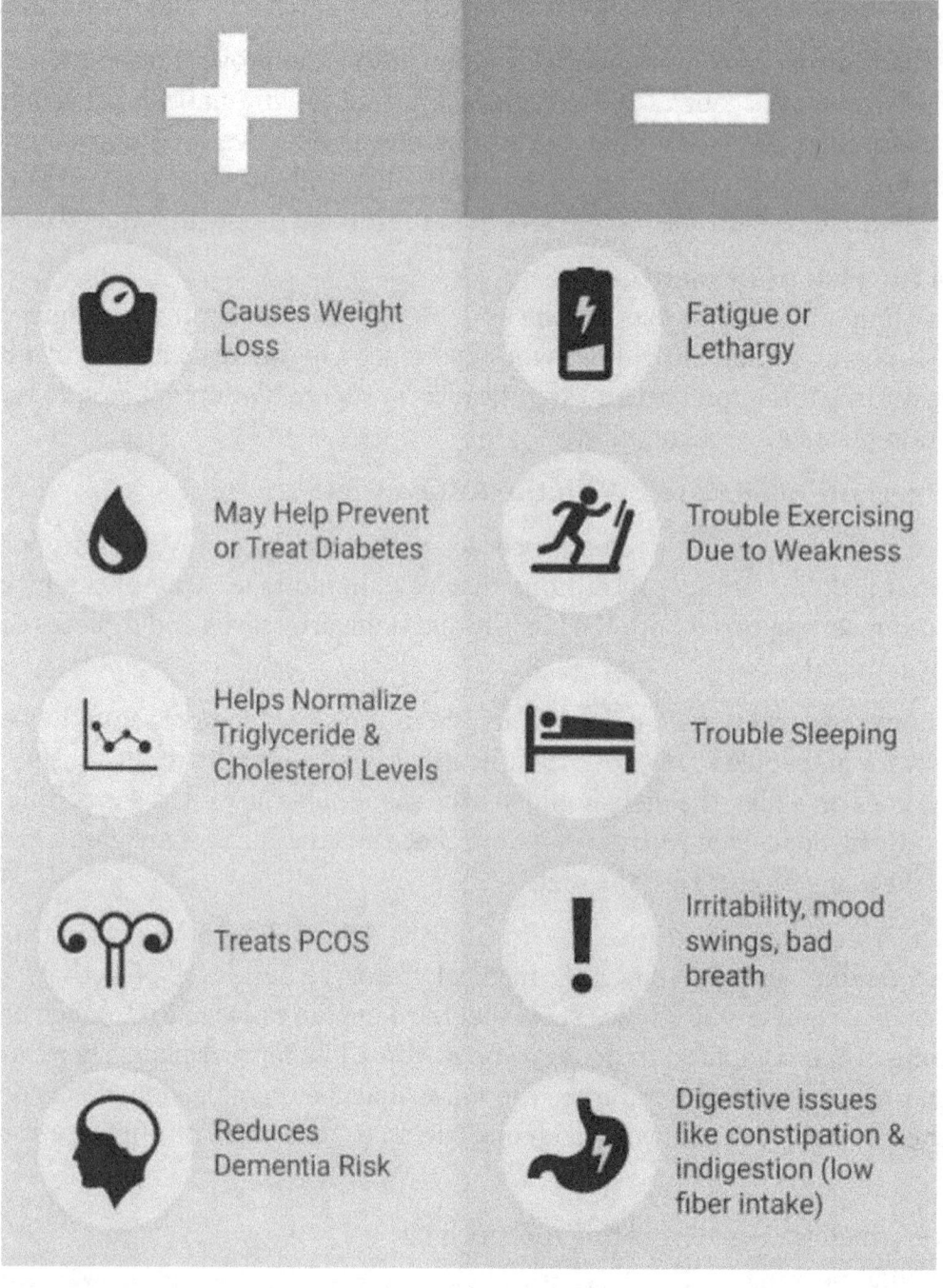

Myths and Facts about the New Atkins Diet

The Atkins diet is one of the most misunderstood programs. For better understanding of what you are getting yourself into, it is important that we address the controversies regarding this diet plan first. Below are common myths about the Atkins diet and the truth behind them.

The Atkins Diet Program does not struggle with excess weight.
The truth is many people have been too obsessed with "low" fat products. They tend to forget that there are two major sources of energy for the body. These are fat and glucose. In truth, fat is completely misunderstood.

This is true: anything in excess is not good for you. It has unhealthy repercussions. However, there are two kinds of fat: the good kind and the bad kind. You cannot simply eradicate fat from your diet because your body needs it, too.

Because of the obsession with "fat", people forget about the other source of energy, glucose derived from carbohydrate foods. When you consume more carbs than your body actually uses, there is a great risk that you will turn them into and store them as fat.

Most weight problems come as a result of issues involving blood sugar and insulin levels. A fat producing hormone, insulin, can make you gain more weight than you intend to. However, if you successfully limit your intake of foods that encourage excessive insulin release, then you have a better chance of getting into your desired shape. The Atkins diet can stabilize your body's insulin level. This way, you can prevent storing more fat than you need in your body.

Atkins dieters only lose water weight, not fat.
It is typical for dieters on any weight loss plan to lose water weight. Atkins dieters lose an enormous amount of weight in the Induction Phase. In the first few days, the weight loss is primarily water, but that is only until ketosis develops. Because of the controlled carbohydrate diet, the body starts to enter a state of ketosis. That is when the magic happens. The body starts to burn body fat because it no longer relies on carbohydrates for energy. At this state and moving forward, dieters burn and lose mainly fat.

It is just a fad.
The Atkins diet program is not just popular because of Hollywood buzz. Celebrities who swear by its effectiveness have undoubtedly been instrumental in getting the word out to the masses about this weight loss solution. It is not just a fad, however. The Atkins diet works by teaching and training your body to burn rather than store fat.

As mentioned previously, the body gets energy through fat and glucose, but the latter is derived mostly from carbohydrates. However, when you limit your intake of carb foods, you force your body to use an alternative source.

Instead of relying on glucose, it will begin to rely on fat— the stored fat, that is. So, stored fat in specific problem areas is accessed for energy. Rather than converting and storing fat, your body starts to rely on fatty acids, burning them for energy. It is a process called ketosis. This results in weight loss.

The Atkins diet does not prohibit you from consuming fat, especially omega-3 fatty acid food sources. However, that does not mean you are free to consume fat to your heart's content. Again, let me emphasize that anything in excess is unhealthy.

The Atkins diet is impossible to maintain because it prohibits carb consumption.
A lot of people think that the Atkins diet does not grant you any access at all to carbohydrates. Low-carb is not no-carb. It is restricted, but this diet is not devoid of carbs. The Atkins diet also does not encourage you to starve yourself to lose weight. Starvation only leads to more intense feelings of hunger. It will spur your appetite out of control; therefore, that kind of strategy for weight loss is one doomed to fail.

Rather, your main objective in the Induction Phase is to use stored fat for energy, and this can only happen when you are in a state of ketosis. Ketosis helps jumpstart the process of weight loss. You can achieve it by reducing your carb consumption. As this phase of the program suggests, your daily carb intake should fall between 18 and 22 grams of net carbs.

For the succeeding phases, you are to increase your carb consumption gradually and slowly reintroduce additional foods that have been prohibited in the first phase.

The Atkins diet will make your body suffer due to lack of nutrients.
Some people are under the impression that the Atkins diet also bans vegetables, fruits, and grains. The first phase of the program prohibits fruits, grains, and high carb vegetables. However, the first phase does not sum up the entire plan. Moreover, although it is restrictive, the Induction Phase is not devoid of nutrients. It does encourage dieters to allot 50 percent of their carb allowance to low carb vegetables including spinach, broccoli, asparagus and other nutrient-dense foods.

As dieters enter the second phase, it is advisable to introduce fruits and other high nutrient foods slowly. Grains will eventually be added along with more fruits and vegetables.

You may lose weight, but you can't maintain it.
This cannot be further from the truth. The Atkins diet consists of four phases, each one leading to the next with a final and unending phase meant to change your eating habits permanently and redo your lifestyle. It is a step-by-step plan offering an excellent variety of meals, so you are filled with satisfaction and motivation to prevent you from going astray from your newly acquired, healthier eating patterns.

Smart Shopping Strategies

These tips will help to turn your grocery shopping excursion into a streamlined and effective experience.

- ✓ **Start with a plan.**

Review your schedule for the week; this will help you determine what meals and snacks you need to shop for. For example, if you know you have an afternoon full of pickups and drop-offs for kids' afterschool activities, pick a recipe that uses a slow cooker so that you have an appetizing low-carb meal waiting when everyone gets home. If you have a busy day of meetings and you know you'll be eating lunch at your desk, make sure you cook an extra serving or two for dinner the night before, so you can take leftovers to work. If the weather looks nice, pick a meal that you can prepare on the grill.

- ✓ **Make a list.**

This helps you stay focused and avoid impulse buys. Shopping list apps make it a breeze to update your list whenever you need to. Some apps allow you to link your list with family members so everyone can update the list in "real time."

- ✓ **Pick a shopping day.**

Pick a day when you won't be rushed trying to get everything you need and when you will have plenty of time to prep your food for the week.

✓ **Never shop when you're hungry.**
Make sure you're hydrated and have a low-carb snack before you go, so you're not tempted by impulse buys simply because you are starving.

✓ **Shop the perimeter of the store.**
This is where the foods that make up the "foundation" of the Atkins diet are located: fruits, vegetables, dairy products, meat, and fish.

✓ **Steer clear of the center aisles.**
The center aisles usually feature the food you are trying to avoid—the processed stuff that is high in carbs and packed with hidden sugars. I usually need to hit the center aisles only for canned tuna and salmon, canned vegetables, broth and bouillon, spices, oils, and condiments.

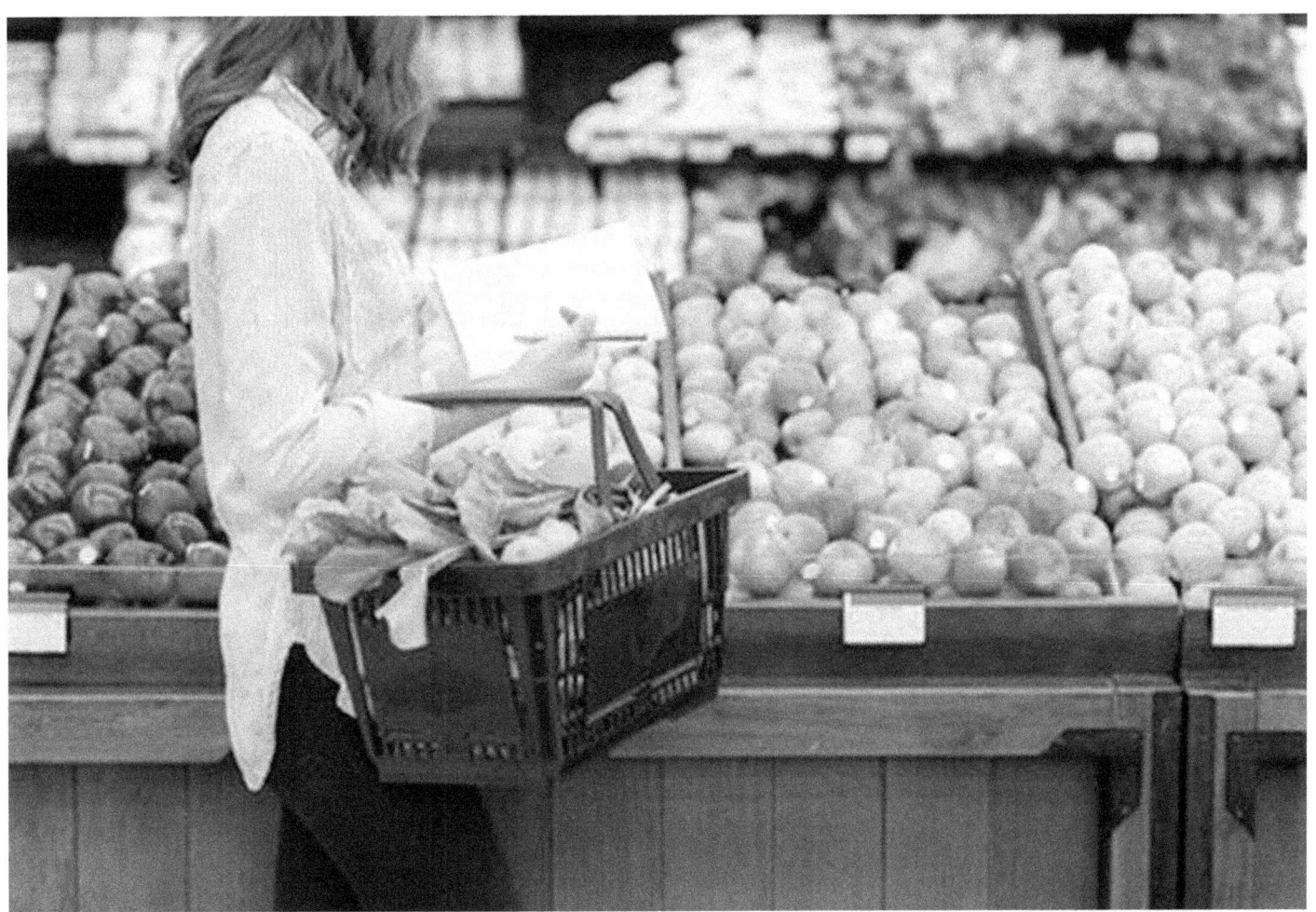

Chapter 2. Three-Week Atkins Meal Plan

Week 1

	Breakfast	Lunch	Snack	Dinner
Monday	Belgian Waffles Page 19	Jalapeño Cheddar Broccoli Soup Page 41	Apple Crumble Page 80	Jerk Chicken Page 62
Tuesday	Birdies in a Basket Page 30	Wedge Salad with Gorgonzola Dressing Page 58	Double Chocolate Brownies Page 81	Mushroom-Herb-Stuffed Chicken Breasts Page 61
Wednesday	Peanut-Strawberry Breakfast Bars Page 22	Cucumber-Dill Salad Page 56	Salted Caramel Cheesecake Bites Page 82	Chicken-Fried Steak Page 64
Thursday	Birdies in a Basket Page 30	Cauliflower Bisque Page 42	Mexican Wedding Cookies Page 83	Roast Beef with Greek Yogurt-Horseradish Sauce Page 63
Friday	Cheese Pancake Page 26	Creamy Cheddar Cheese Soup Page 48	Chocolate-Orange Soufflés Page 75	Salmon with Rosemary Page 73
Saturday	Atkins Yorkshire Pudding Page 29	Spicy Korean Soup with Scallions Page 43	Mini-Muffin-Tin Chocolate Brownies Page 78	Year-Round Barbecued Brisket Page 72
Sunday	Cranberry-Orange Loaf Page 27	Athenian Salad Page 51	Cranberry-Orange Fool Page 77	Baked Salmon with Mustard-Nut Crust Page 69

Week 2

	Breakfast	**Lunch**	**Snack**	**Dinner**
Monday	Broiler Huevos Rancheros Page 25	Tomato and Red Onion Salad Page 60	Mini-Muffin-Tin Chocolate Brownies Page 78	Beef Bourguignon Page 70
Tuesday	Pancakes With Ricotta-Apricot Filling Page 28	Caprese Salad Page 52	Apple Crumble Page 80	Fontina-and-Prosciutto-Stuffed Veal Chops Page 66
Wednesday	Whole-Wheat Currant Scones Page 21	Slaw with Vinegar Dressing Page 57	Double Chocolate Brownies Page 81	Baked Bluefish with Garlic and Lime Page 68
Thursday	Flaxseed Pancake Page 20	Watercress Bacon Salad with Ranch Dressing Page 54	Salted Caramel Cheesecake Bites Page 82	Fontina-and-Prosciutto-Stuffed Veal Chops Page 66
Friday	Belgian Waffles Page 19	Cold Roasted Tomato Soup Page 50	Mexican Wedding Cookies Page 83	Chicken-Fried Steak Page 64
Saturday	Birdies in a Basket Page 30	Cream of Broccoli Soup Page 49	Chocolate-Orange Soufflés Page 75	Mushroom-Herb-Stuffed Chicken Breasts Page 61
Sunday	Peanut-Strawberry Breakfast Bars Page 22	Old Bay Shrimp Salad Page 53	Mexican Wedding Cookies Page 83	Chicken-Fried Steak Page 64

Week 3

	Breakfast	**Lunch**	**Snack**	**Dinner**
Monday	Crunchy Tropical Berry and Almond Breakfast Parfait Page 23	Caprese Salad Page 52	Salted Caramel Cheesecake Bites Page 82	Year-Round Barbecued Brisket Page 72
Tuesday	Broiler Huevos Rancheros Page 25	Creamy Cheddar Cheese Soup Page 47	Chocolate-Orange Soufflés Page 75	Beef Bourguignon Page 70
Wednesday	Pancakes With Ricotta-Apricot Filling Page 28	Slaw with Vinegar Dressing Page 57	Salted Caramel Cheesecake Bites Page 82	Fontina-and-Prosciutto-Stuffed Veal Chops Page 66
Thursday	Whole-Wheat Currant Scones Page 21	Spicy Korean Soup with Scallions Page 42	Mexican Wedding Cookies Page 83	Baked Bluefish with Garlic and Lime Page 68
Friday	Flaxseed Pancake Page 20	Tomato and Red Onion Salad Page 59	Cranberry-Orange Fool Page 77	Fontina-and-Prosciutto-Stuffed Veal Chops Page 66
Saturday	Atkins Yorkshire Pudding Page 29	Watercress Bacon Salad with Ranch Dressing Page 54	Mini-Muffin-Tin Chocolate Brownies Page 78	Jerk Chicken Page 62
Sunday	Cauliflower Rice Scrambles Page 24	Wedge Salad with Gorgonzola Dressing Page 57	Mini-Muffin-Tin Chocolate Brownies Page 78	Mushroom-Herb-Stuffed Chicken Breasts Page 61

Chapter 3. Recipes
BREAKFAST
Belgian Waffles

Prep time: 10 minutes

Cooking time: 10 minutes

Servings: 8

Nutrients per serving:

Carbohydrates – 4 g

Net Carbs – 2.4 g

Fat – 6 g

Protein – 3 g

Calories – 112

Ingredients:

- 1 cup bake mix
- 1 Tbsp baking powder
- 3 packets sugar substitute
- 1 tsp salt
- ¼ cup heavy cream
- 3 eggs
- 1 tsp vanilla
- ½ cup ice water

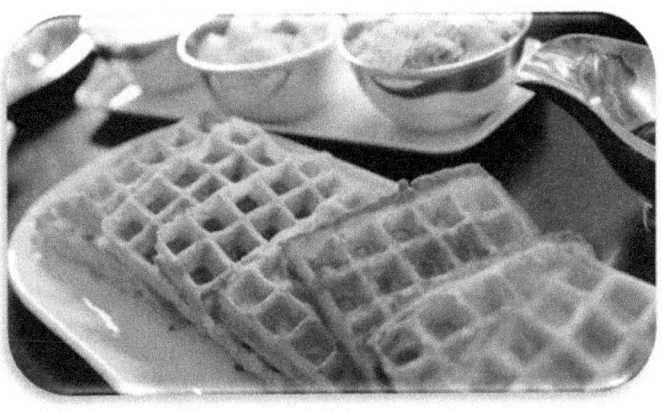

Instructions:

1. Heat a waffle iron. Whisk together the bake mix, baking powder, sugar substitute and salt. Add cream, eggs, vanilla extract and ice water. Pour in a little more water if necessary, 1 tablespoon at a time, until batter spreads easily.
2. Place approximately 3 tablespoons batter in center of waffle iron. Cook according to manufacturer's directions until crisp and dark golden brown. Repeat with remaining batter.

Flaxseed Pancake

Prep time: 10 minutes

Cooking time: 10 minutes

Servings: 2

Nutrients per serving:

Carbohydrates – 3.6 g

Net Carbs – 2 g

Fat – 6.8 g

Protein – 16.5 g

Calories – 213

Ingredients:

- 1 pinch cinnamon
- 1 tsp vanilla
- 2 tsp baking powder
- 6 Tbsp ground flax seed
- 1 cup egg beaters

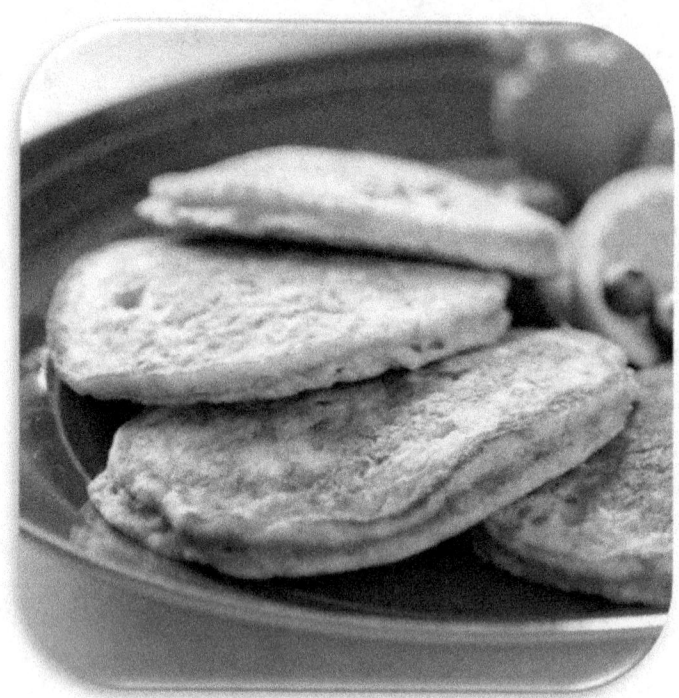

Instructions:

1. Pour egg beaters into a bowl.
2. Add the remaining ingredients into the bowl. Mix well.
3. Set aside for 1 minute then mix again.
4. Put a skillet over medium heat and spray with oil.
5. Divide pancake mixture into four batches. Cook each batch as you would a regular pancake.

Whole-Wheat Currant Scones

Prep time: 20 minutes

Cooking time: 10 minutes

Servings: 12

Nutrients per serving:

Carbohydrates – 14 g

Net Carbs – 10.4 g

Fat – 12 g

Protein – 8 g

Calories – 190

Ingredients:

- ¼ cup currants
- 1 cup whole-wheat flour
- 1 cup Atkins Cuisine All Purpose Baking Mix
- 2 Tbsp granular sugar substitute
- 4 tsp baking powder
- 2 tsp ground ginger
- ⅛ tsp ground nutmeg
- ⅛ tsp salt
- 5 Tbsp cold unsalted butter, cut into pieces
- 2 large eggs, lightly beaten
- ¾ cup heavy cream

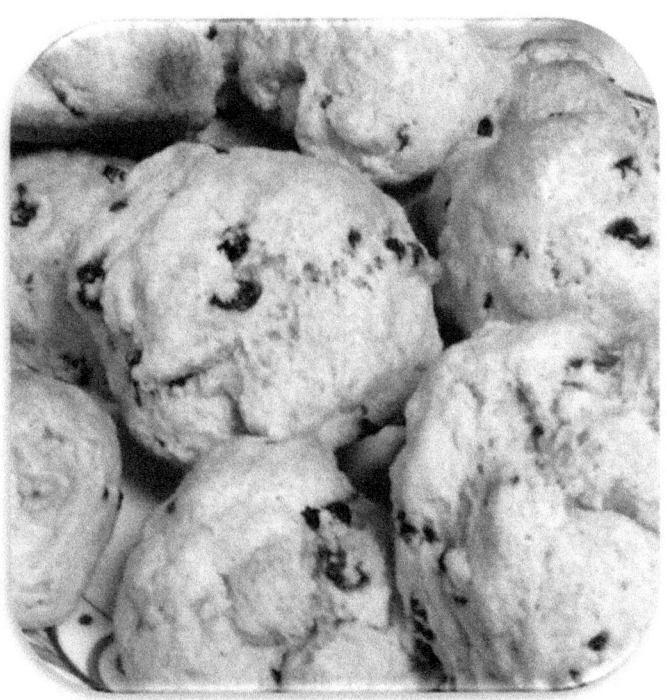

Instructions:

1. Heat oven to 400°F. Soak currants for 15 minutes in a cup of warm water.
2. Pulse flour, baking mix, sugar substitute, baking powder, ginger, nutmeg, and salt in a food processor. Add butter; pulse until well combined. Add eggs and heavy cream; pulse for 2 minutes. Drain currants and add; pulse until just combined.
3. Drop ¼-cup mounds on an ungreased baking sheet; press gently to flatten slightly. Bake until lightly golden, about 10 minutes. Serve warm or at room temperature.

Peanut-Strawberry Breakfast Bars

Prep time: 15 minutes

Cooking time: 25 minutes

Servings: 12

Nutrients per serving:

Carbohydrates – 17 g

Net Carbs – 12 g

Fat – 18 g

Protein – 10 g

Calories – 270

Ingredients:

- Olive oil cooking spray
- 1¼ cups old-fashioned rolled oats
- 1¼ cups granular sugar substitute
- ½ cup all purpose baking mix
- ¼ cup whole-wheat flour
- ¼ tsp salt
- ½ cup (1 stick) unsalted butter, melted
- 3 large eggs, lightly beaten
- ¾ cup unsweetened natural peanut butter
- ½ cup no-sugar-added strawberry jam

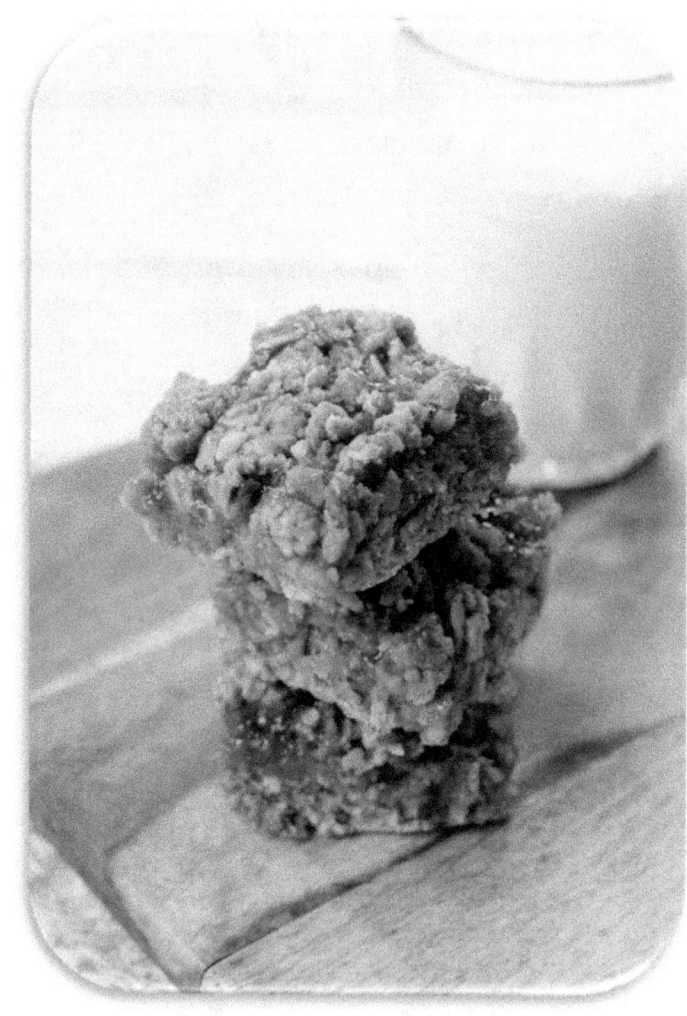

Instructions:

1. Heat oven to 350°F. Mist a 7-by-11-inch baking dish with cooking spray.
2. Mix oats, sugar substitute, baking mix, flour, and salt in a medium bowl; stir in butter and eggs until well combined. Spread out half the dough in the baking dish. Spread peanut butter evenly over dough; spread preserves evenly over peanut butter. Crumble remaining dough over preserves.
3. Bake for about 25 minutes. Cool completely before cutting into 12 pieces.

Crunchy Tropical Berry and Almond Breakfast Parfait

Prep time: 10 minutes

Cooking time: 10 minutes

Servings: 4

Nutrients per serving:

Carbohydrates – 14 g

Net Carbs – 8 g

Fat – 21 g

Protein – 6 g

Calories – 260

Ingredients:

- ½ cup heavy cream
- 1½ tsp granular sugar substitute, divided
- ¼ tsp coconut extract or pure vanilla extract
- ½ cup plain unsweetened whole-milk Greek yogurt
- 1 cup raspberries
- 1 cup blueberries or sliced strawberries
- 8 Tbsp Sweet and Salty Almonds
- ½ cup unsweetened shredded coconut, toasted

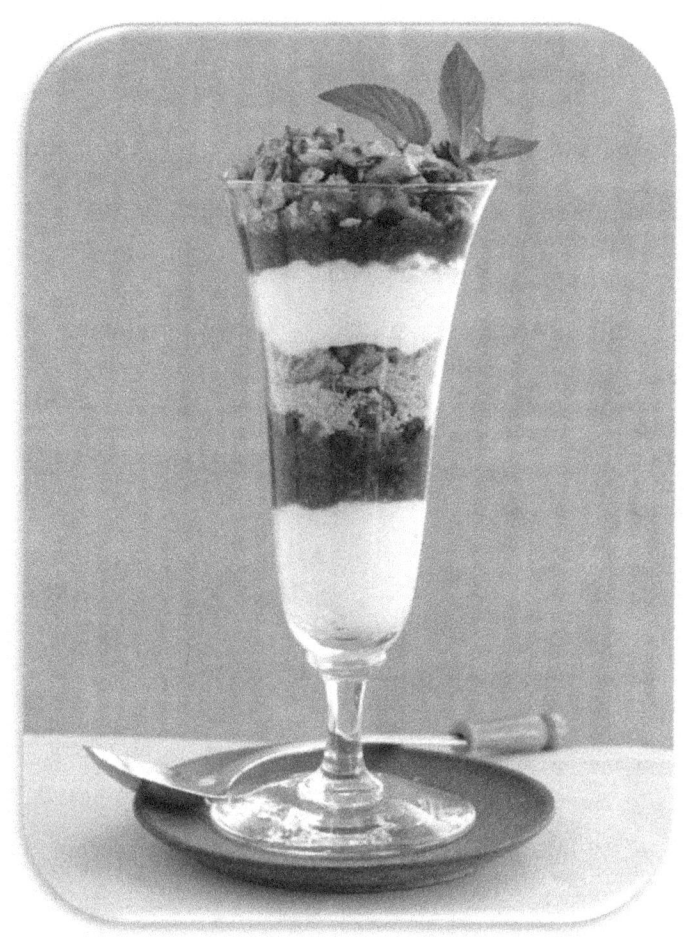

Instructions:

1. Combine cream, ½ tsp sugar substitute, and coconut extract or vanilla extract in a medium bowl; whip with an electric mixer for 3 minutes. Add in the yogurt.
2. Mix raspberries and remaining sugar substitute in a blender until smooth.
3. In 4 parfait glasses, alternate layers of whipped cream, raspberry purée, blueberries, nuts, and shredded coconut, making two layers of each. Serve right away.

Cauliflower Rice Scrambles

Prep time: 10 minutes

Cooking time: 15 minutes

Servings: 4

Nutrients per serving:

Carbohydrates – 8.4 g

Net Carbs – 5.1 g

Fat – 26.2 g

Protein – 28.1 g

Calories – 381

Ingredients:

- 1 head cauliflower, cut into florets (about 5 cups)
- 8 slices bacon
- 2 jalapeños, seeded and diced
- 8 large eggs
- 1 cup shredded cheddar cheese
- Hot sauce, to taste

Instructions:

1. Chop the cauliflower florets roughly in a food processor.
2. Warm the bacon in a large skillet over medium heat, and cook 4 to 5 minutes, stirring occasionally. Transfer to a plate. Do not discard the bacon grease.
3. Add the cauliflower and jalapeños to the bacon grease in the skillet, and cook 5 to 6 minutes, stirring often, until the cauliflower is soft.
4. Place the eggs and cheddar in a large bowl, and gently whisk. Add the eggs to the skillet and cook 3 to 4 minutes, stirring occasionally, until firm. Serve immediately with the bacon and hot sauce, if desired.

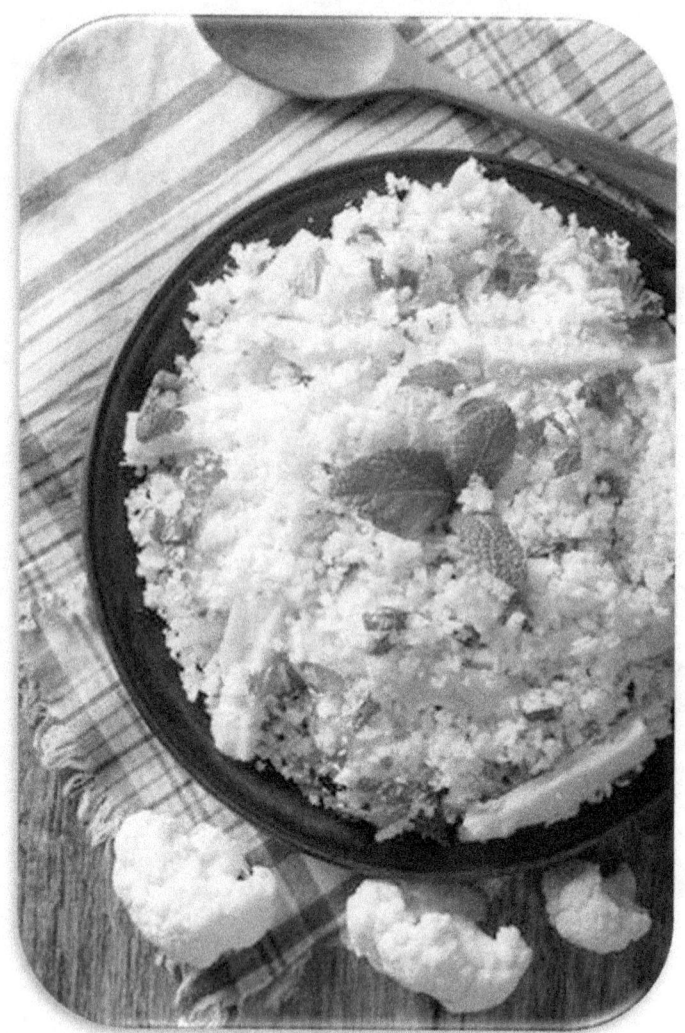

Broiler Huevos Rancheros

Prep time: 15 minutes

Cooking time: 5 minutes

Servings: 4

Nutrients per serving:

Carbohydrates – 16.6 g

Net Carbs – 9 g

Fat – 27.2 g

Protein – 23.6 g

Calories – 396

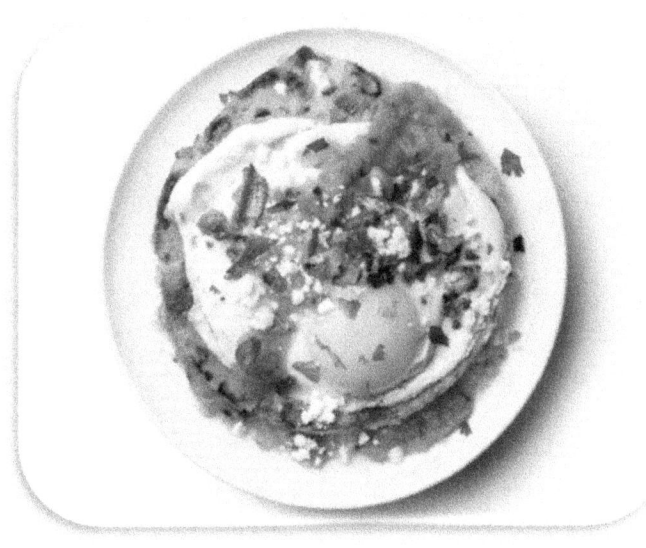

Ingredients:

- Olive oil spray
- 2 chorizo sausage links, (about 6 ounces) thinly sliced
- 1 bunch asparagus, trimmed and chopped
- 2 cups broccoli florets
- 2 cups cauliflower florets
- 8 large eggs
- ½ cup commercial tomato salsa
- 1 ripe Hass avocado, cut into wedges
- ¼ cup sour cream

Instructions:

1. Set the oven to broil and coat a large skillet with olive oil spray. Place over medium heat and add the chorizo, browning for 3 to 4 minutes, stirring well, until it renders its fat. Add the asparagus, broccoli, and cauliflower, and cook 3 to 4 minutes, until the vegetables start to soften. Crack the eggs on top.
2. Cook under the broiler on the middle oven rack for 3 to 4 minutes. Serve immediately with the salsa, avocado, and sour cream.

Cheese Pancake

Prep time: 15 minutes

Cooking time: 3 minutes

Servings: 4

Nutrients per serving:

Carbohydrates – 2 g

Net Carbs – 0.8 g

Fat – 26.4 g

Protein – 11.1 g

Calories – 231

Ingredients:

- 1 Tbsp ground flax seed
- ½ tsp ground cinnamon
- 1 packet Stevia
- 4 oz cream cheese
- 2 eggs

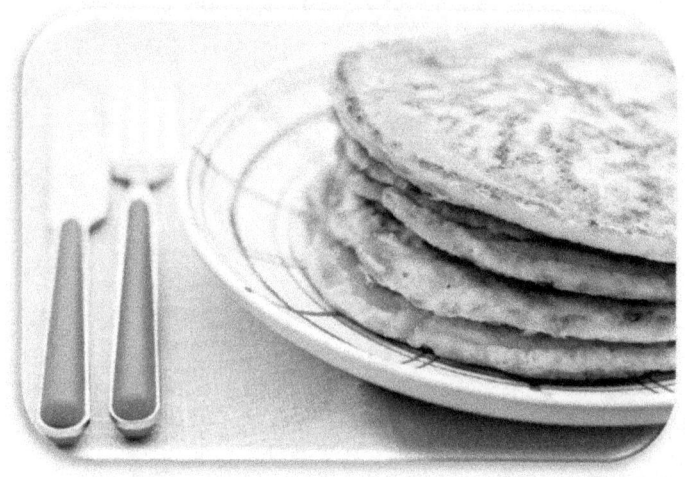

Instructions:

1. Whisk the egg whites in a bowl.
2. In a separate bowl, beat the cream cheese with an electric mixer until smooth.
3. Combine the egg yolk with the cream cheese. Add the flax seed, salt, stevia and cinnamon. Continue to beat the mixture.
4. Fold in the beaten egg whites.
5. Put a pan over medium heat and add a small amount of butter.
6. Scoop ¼ cup from the mixture.
7. Cook the pancake for 3 minutes or until golden brown. Then, serve.

Cranberry-Orange Loaf

Prep time: 20 minutes

Cooking time: 50 minutes

Servings: 5

Nutrients per serving:

Carbohydrates – 4 g

Net Carbs – 2.5 g

Fat – 8 g

Protein – 2 g

Calories – 106

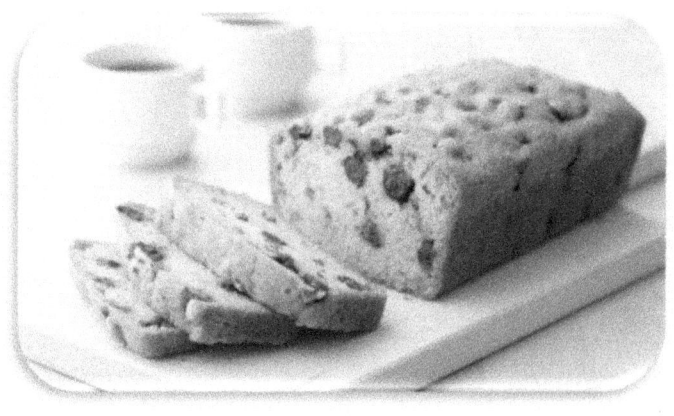

Ingredients:

- 1 cup fresh or frozen cranberries, thawed
- 1¼ cups Atkins Bake Mix
- ½ cup walnuts, toasted and ground
- 16 packets sugar substitute
- 1 tsp baking soda
- ½ tsp salt
- 1 stick (8 Tbsp) butter, softened
- 2 Tbsp sour cream
- 2 eggs
- 1 Tbsp grated fresh orange zest
- 1 tsp vanilla extract
- 2 egg whites

Instructions:

1. Heat oven to 350°F Grease a 9-inch-by-5-inch loaf pan; set aside. Coarsely chop cranberries; set aside. In a medium bowl, mix walnuts, sugar substitute, bake mix, baking soda and salt until combined.
2. In another bowl, beat butter 3 minutes with an electric mixer on medium, until fluffy. Beat in sour cream, eggs, orange zest and vanilla extract. Fold in cranberries.
3. Combine together the bake mix mixture and butter mixture. In another bowl, beat egg whites for about 2 minutes. In three portions, fold egg whites into batter.
4. Spoon batter into prepared pan. Bake 50 to 55 minutes. Cool on wire rack. Cut loaf into thin slices.

Pancakes With Ricotta-Apricot Filling

Prep time: 15 minutes

Cooking time: 20 minutes

Servings: 4

Nutrients per serving:

Carbohydrates – 3 g

Net Carbs – 3 g

Fat – 5.5 g

Protein – 3 g

Calories – 76

Ingredients:

- 3 eggs
- 3 Tbsp Atkins Bake Mix
- ¼ tsp salt
- ⅓ cup heavy cream;
- ¾ cup ricotta cheese
- ¼ cup sugar-free apricot jam
- 1 packet sugar substitute
- 1½ Tbsp butter

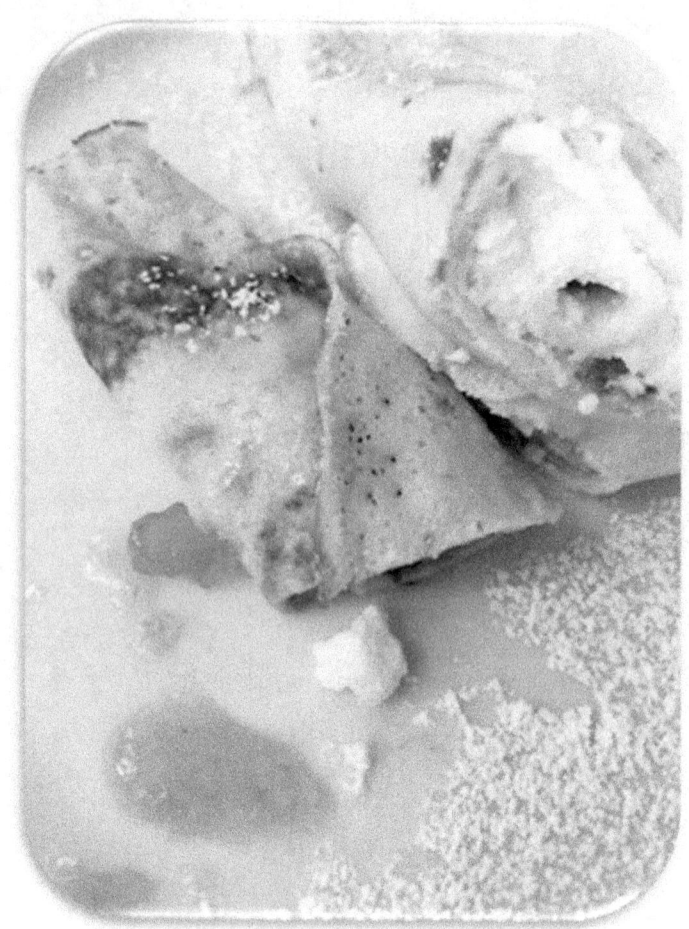

Instructions:

1. In a bowl, whisk eggs, bake mix and salt until smooth. Gradually whisk in cream. Set aside for 5 minutes.
2. Press ricotta through a fine sieve into a bowl. Mix in jam and sugar substitute.
3. Melt butter in a nonstick skillet over medium heat. Pour in 2 tablespoons batter and tilt skillet to coat bottom. Cook until golden on bottom; turn over. Cook 1 minute more. Transfer to a plate. Repeat with remaining batter.
4. Spread pancakes with ricotta mixture, roll up and serve.

Atkins Yorkshire Pudding

Prep time: 5 minutes

Cooking time: 35 minutes

Servings: 9

Nutrients per serving:

Carbohydrates – 5 g

Net Carbs – 4 g

Fat – 11 g

Protein – 5 g

Calories – 149

Ingredients:

- ½ cup Atkins Bake Mix
- ¼ cup wheat gluten
- 3 eggs
- 1 cup whole milk
- 1 tsp salt
- ⅓ cup beef drippings or vegetable oil

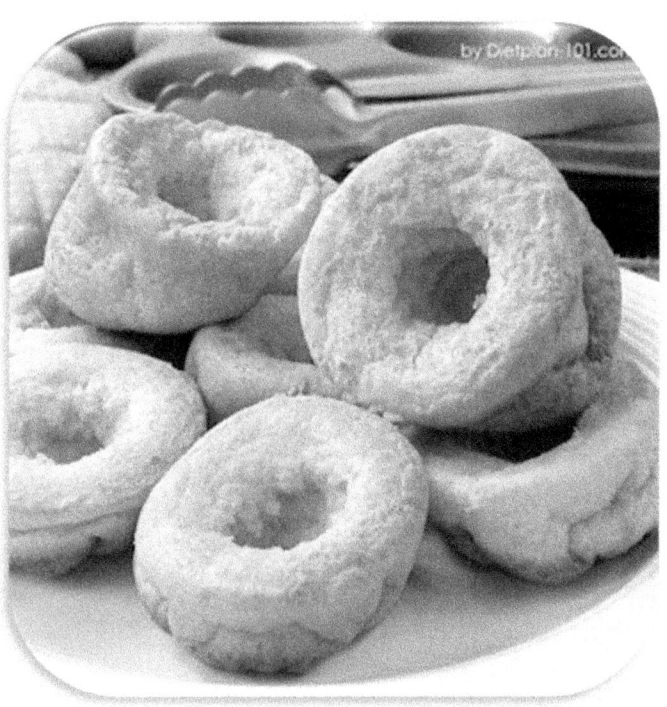

Instructions:

1. Heat oven to 450°F. Whisk together bake mix, gluten, eggs, milk and salt.
2. Pour drippings or oil into an muffin tin (½ tbsp each); place on center rack in oven for 10 minutes, until smoky hot. Add batter; bake 15 minutes. Lower temperature to 350°F; cook 20 minutes more, until lightly browned. Serve warm.

Birdies in a Basket

Prep time: 20 minutes

Cooking time: 35 minutes

Servings: 4

Nutrients per serving:

Carbohydrates – 8.8 g

Net Carbs – 6 g

Fat – 27.3 g

Protein – 21.6 g

Calories – 362

Ingredients:

- 1 Tbsp olive oil
- ½ bunch asparagus, trimmed and sliced
- ½ tsp seasoning salt
- 2 large green bell peppers, halved crosswise, seeded
- 4 large eggs
- 2 cups shredded cheddar cheese

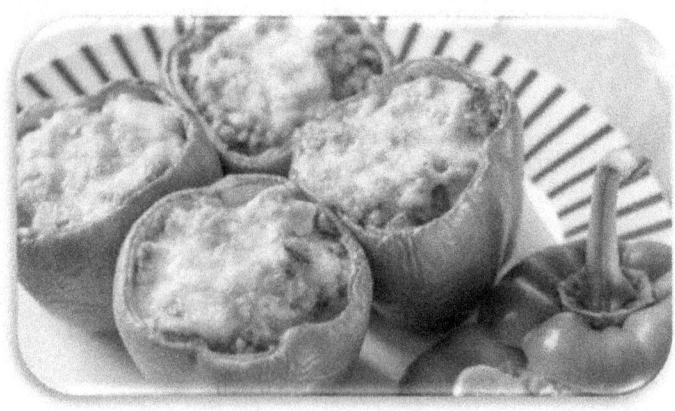

Instructions:

1. Heat a skillet, and add the olive oil. Add the asparagus and seasoning salt; cook 3 to 4 minutes, until the asparagus softens. Transfer to a plate.
2. Preheat the oven to 350°F. Place the peppers in the skillet, stem side down, and sear for 1 minute over medium heat. Flip and crack an egg into each pepper half. Top with the asparagus and sprinkle with the cheddar.
3. Bake for 30 minutes, the whites of the eggs are cooked through. Serve immediately.

VEGETABLES AND OTHER SIDES

Sautéed Greens with Pecans

Prep time: 20 minutes

Cooking time: 10 minutes

Servings: 4

Nutrients per serving:

Carbohydrates – 6 g

Net Carbs – 3 g

Fat – 10 g

Protein – 3 g

Calories – 120

Ingredients:

- 1 (1-pound) bunch Swiss chard or mustard, beet, or turnip greens
- 1 Tbsp extra-virgin olive oil
- 2 cloves garlic, chopped
- ⅓ cup pecans, toasted and coarsely chopped
- ½ tsp salt
- ⅛ tsp freshly ground black pepper

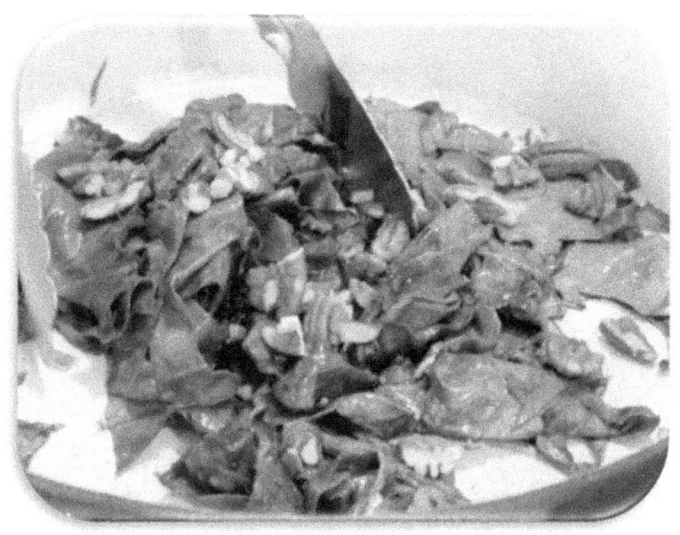

Instructions:

1. Chop the leaves of the greens crosswise into 1-inch slices; cut stems into ½-inch pieces. Rinse thoroughly.
2. Bring a pot of salted water to a boil over high heat. Add stems, reduce heat to medium-low, and simmer 2 minutes; add leaves and cook until stems are tender, about 3 minutes longer. Drain.
3. In a skillet, heat the oil over high heat. Add garlic and sauté until fragrant, about 30 seconds. Add greens, pecans, salt, and pepper; sauté to heat through, about 2 minutes. Serve hot.

Stir-Fried Broccolini with Cashews

Prep time: 20 minutes

Cooking time: 20 minutes

Servings: 4

Nutrients per serving:

Carbohydrates – 10 g

Net Carbs – 7 g

Fat – 11 g

Protein – 5 g

Calories – 150

Ingredients:

- 2 Tbsp canola oil
- 1 scallion, thinly sliced
- 2 tsp peeled and minced fresh ginger
- 2 cloves garlic, minced
- 2 bunches Broccolini
- ¾ cup water
- ¼ cup cashews, toasted and chopped
- 3 Tbsp tamari
- ¼ tsp red pepper flakes
- ⅛ tsp dark (toasted) sesame oil

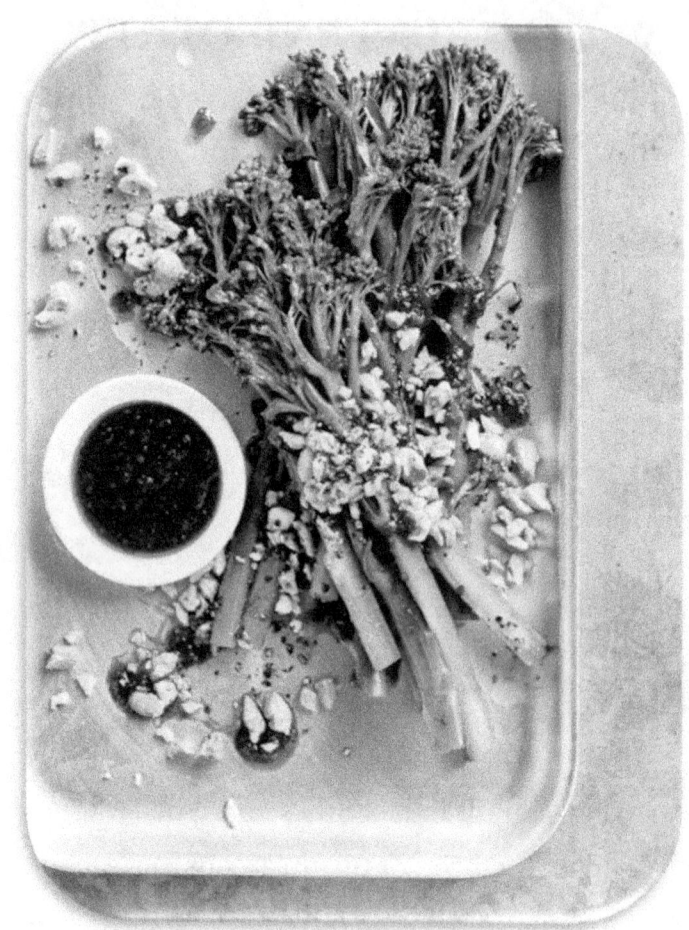

Instructions:

1. Heat the canola oil in a wok. Add scallion, ginger, and garlic; sauté until fragrant, stirring constantly, about 45 seconds.
2. Add Broccolini and water; simmer for about 2–3 minutes.
3. Add in cashews, tamari, and red pepper flakes; cook for about 1 minute. Stir in sesame oil and serve.

Roasted Lemon-Garlic Brussels Sprouts

Prep time: 10 minutes

Cooking time: 20 minutes

Servings: 6

Nutrients per serving:

Carbohydrates – 9 g

Net Carbs – 5 g

Fat – 12 g

Protein – 3 g

Calories – 150

Ingredients:

- 2 (10-ounce) containers Brussels sprouts, trimmed and halved
- 5 Tbsp virgin olive oil
- 1 Tbsp freshly grated lemon zest
- 2 cloves garlic, chopped
- 1 tsp chopped fresh thyme
- 1 tsp salt
- ¼ tsp freshly ground black pepper

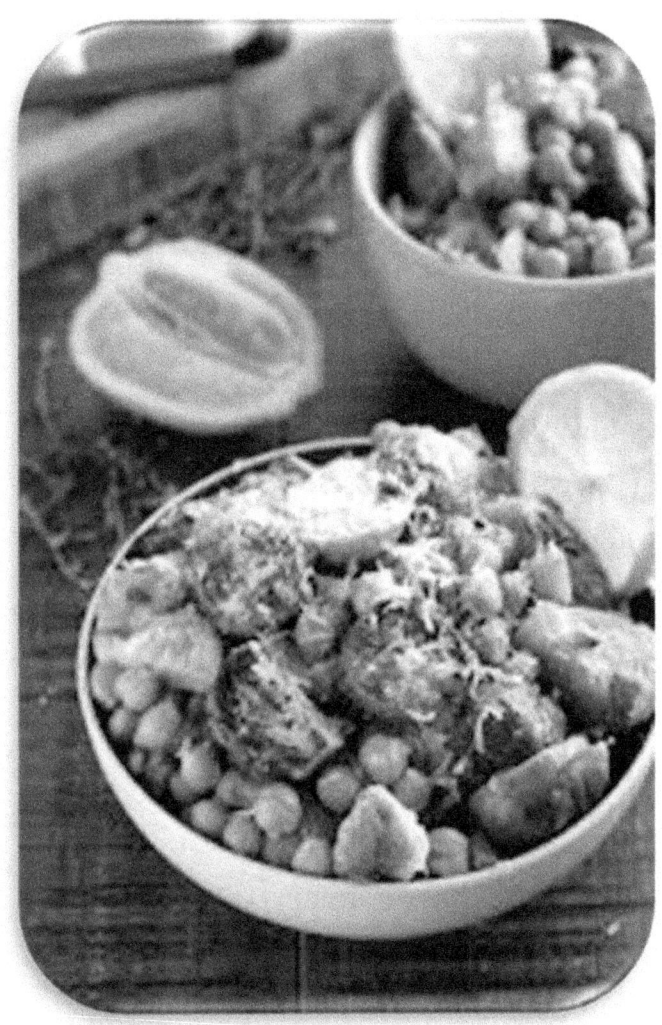

Instructions:

1. Heat oven to 375°F.
2. Combine sprouts, oil, lemon zest, garlic, thyme, salt, and pepper in a large jelly-roll pan or shallow baking dish; toss well. Arrange sprouts in a single layer; roast, stirring occasionally, until tender and light brown, about 20 minutes. Serve hot.

Sautéed Baby Bok Choy with Garlic and Lemon Zest

Prep time: 10 minutes

Cooking time: 3 minutes

Servings: 6

Nutrients per serving:

Carbohydrates – 1 g

Net Carbs – 1 g

Fat – 5 g

Protein – 1 g

Calories – 45

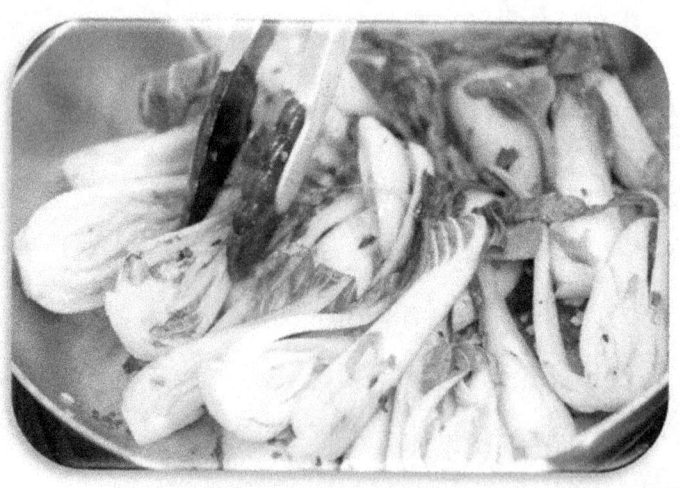

Ingredients:

- 2 Tbsp virgin olive oil
- 2 cloves garlic, chopped
- 2 tsp freshly grated lemon zest
- 18 heads baby bok choy, trimmed, heads cut in half lengthwise
- ¼ tsp salt
- ⅛ tsp freshly ground black pepper

Instructions:

1. Heat oil in a skillet. Add garlic and lemon zest and sauté until fragrant, about 30 seconds.
2. Add bok choy, salt, and pepper; sauté until just wilted, about 2 minutes. Serve hot.

Swiss Chard with Pine Nuts

Prep time: 10 minutes
Cooking time: 10 minutes
Servings: 6

Nutrients per serving:

Carbohydrates – 4 g

Net Carbs – 3 g

Fat – 8 g

Protein – 2 g

Calories – 90

Ingredients:

- 1 (1- to 1¼-pound) bunch Swiss chard, leaves and stems separated
- 2 Tbsp virgin olive oil
- 1 clove garlic, chopped
- ½ tsp salt
- ¼ tsp freshly ground black pepper
- 3 Tbsp pine nuts, toasted

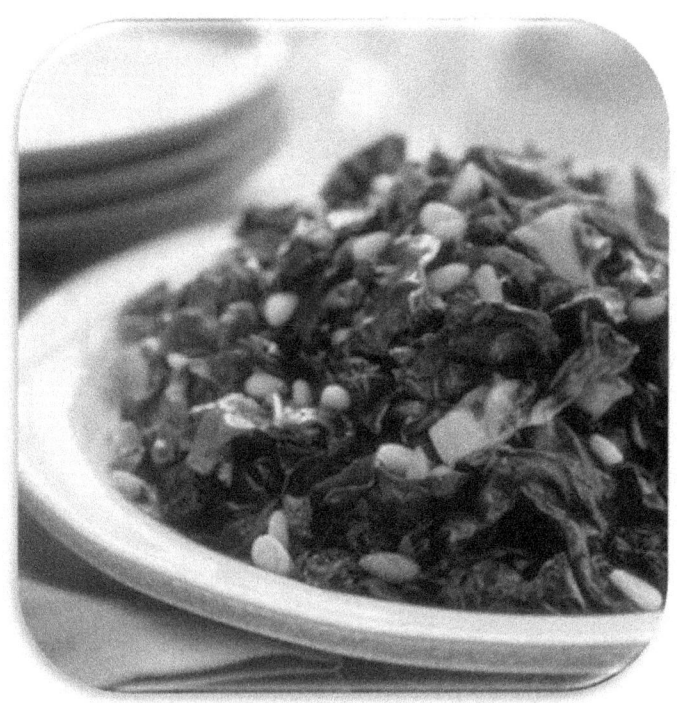

Instructions:

1. Chop chard leaves crosswise into 2-inch slices; cut stems into ½-inch pieces. Rinse thoroughly, then spin dry.
2. Heat oil in a saucepan over high heat. Add garlic and sauté until fragrant, about 30 seconds. Add chard stems, salt and pepper; sauté until stems are almost tender, about 5 minutes. Add chard leaves and sauté until chard is completely tender, about 5 minutes. Stir in pine nuts and serve.

Braised Lettuce

Prep time: 10 minutes
Cooking time: 10 minutes
Servings: 6

Nutrients per serving:

Carbohydrates – 4 g

Net Carbs – 3 g

Fat – 8 g

Protein – 2 g

Calories – 90

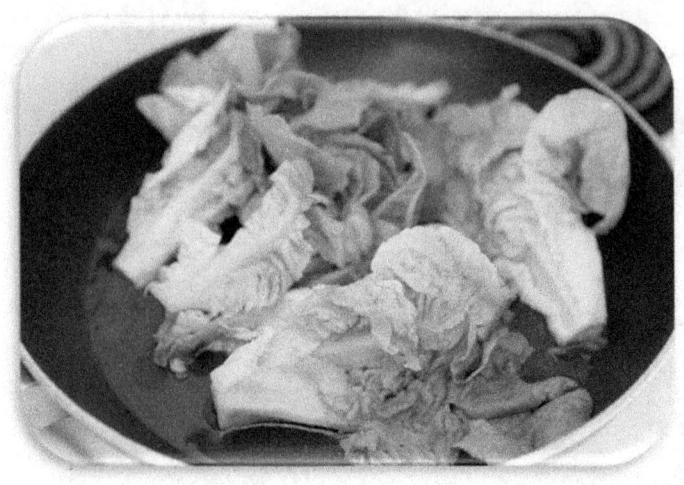

Ingredients:

- 2 Tbsp butter
- 1 clove garlic, chopped
- 2 heads Boston or Bibb lettuce, halved lengthwise, rinsed well, and patted dry
- ½ cup chicken broth
- ¼ tsp salt
- ⅛ tsp freshly ground black pepper
- 2 Tbsp heavy cream

Instructions:

1. Melt butter in a skillet. Add garlic and sauté until fragrant, about 30 seconds. Add lettuce, cut side down, and cook 2 minutes. Turn lettuce over; add broth, salt, and pepper. Cover and simmer until lettuce is slightly wilted, about 3 minutes.
2. Add cream and simmer, uncovered, until liquid is reduced by half, about 5 minutes. Serve right away.

Roasted Cauliflower

Prep time: 15 minutes
Cooking time: 30 minutes
Servings: 4

Nutrients per serving:

Carbohydrates – 11 g

Net Carbs – 7 g

Fat – 11 g

Protein – 3 g

Calories – 150

Ingredients:

- 1 head cauliflower, broken into florets and cut into ⅓-inch slices
- 2 small yellow or white onions, cut into wedges
- 3 Tbsp virgin olive oil
- ¾ tsp salt, divided
- ¼ tsp freshly ground black pepper, divided

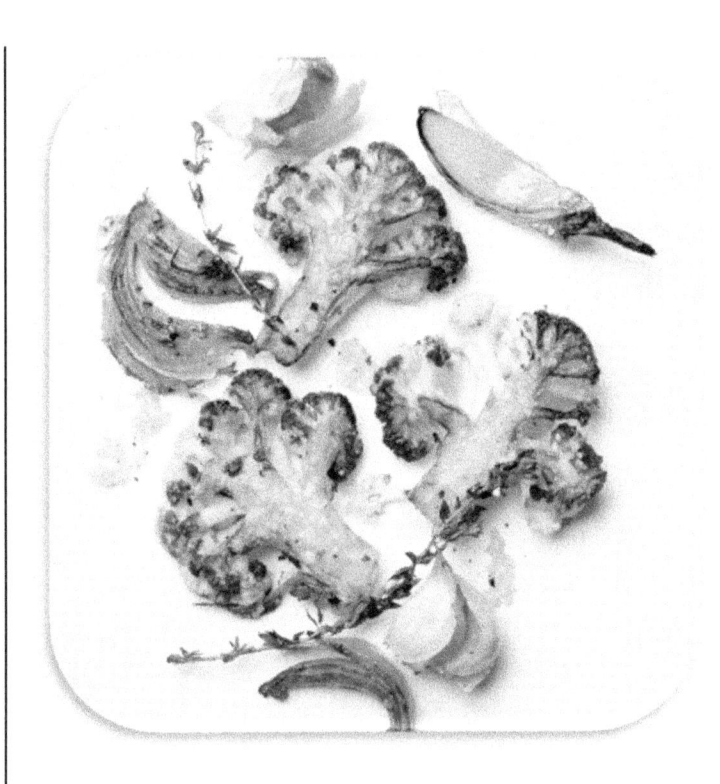

Instructions:

1. Heat oven to 450°F.
2. Combine cauliflower, onions, oil, salt, and pepper in a large jelly-roll pan or shallow baking dish; toss well. Arrange in a single layer, then roast for about 30 minutes. Serve warm.

Sautéed Spinach with Caramelized Shallots

Prep time: 15 minutes

Cooking time: 15 minutes

Servings: 6

Nutrients per serving:

Carbohydrates – 4.4 g

Net Carbs – 2.8 g

Fat – 4.5 g

Protein – 2.4 g

Calories – 62

Ingredients:

- 1 Tbsp unsalted butter
- 1 Tbsp olive oil
- 3 shallots, thinly sliced (about ⅓ cup)
- ¼ tsp salt
- ¼ tsp freshly ground black pepper
- ¼ tsp stevia, optional
- Olive oil spray
- 1 pound baby spinach or baby kale

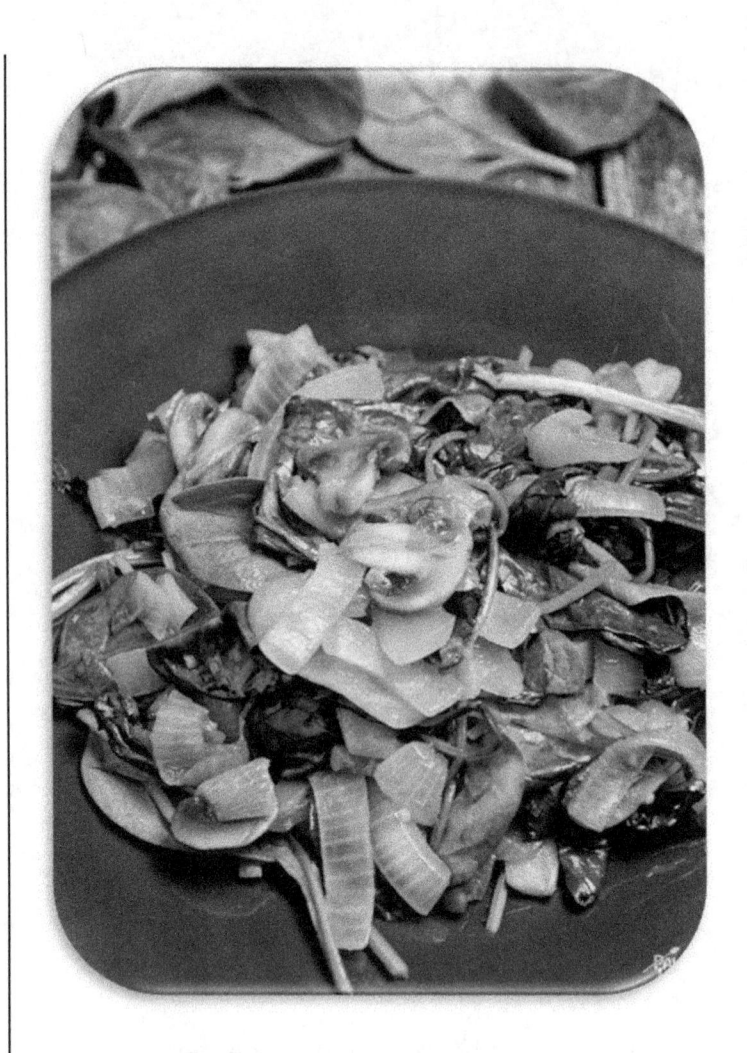

Instructions:

1. Warm the butter and olive oil in a small skillet over medium heat. Add the shallots, salt, black pepper, and stevia. Cook for about 12 minutes, adding 1 to 2 tablespoons of water if the shallots stick. Transfer the shallots to a plate.
2. Coat the skillet with the olive oil spray and, working in batches, add the spinach; cook 1 to 2 minutes. Top with the shallots, and serve immediately.

Shishito Peppers with Hot Paprika Mayonnaise

Prep time: 15 minutes

Cooking time: 3 minutes

Servings: 4

Nutrients per serving:

Carbohydrates – 7.1 g

Net Carbs – 2.7 g

Fat – 23.7 g

Protein – 2.2 g

Calories – 245

Ingredients:

- 4 quarts shishito peppers (about 48)
- ½ cup mayonnaise
- Zest of 1 lemon, finely grated
- 1 Tbsp tomato paste
- 1 Tbsp hot paprika
- 1 Tbsp grape seed or coconut oil

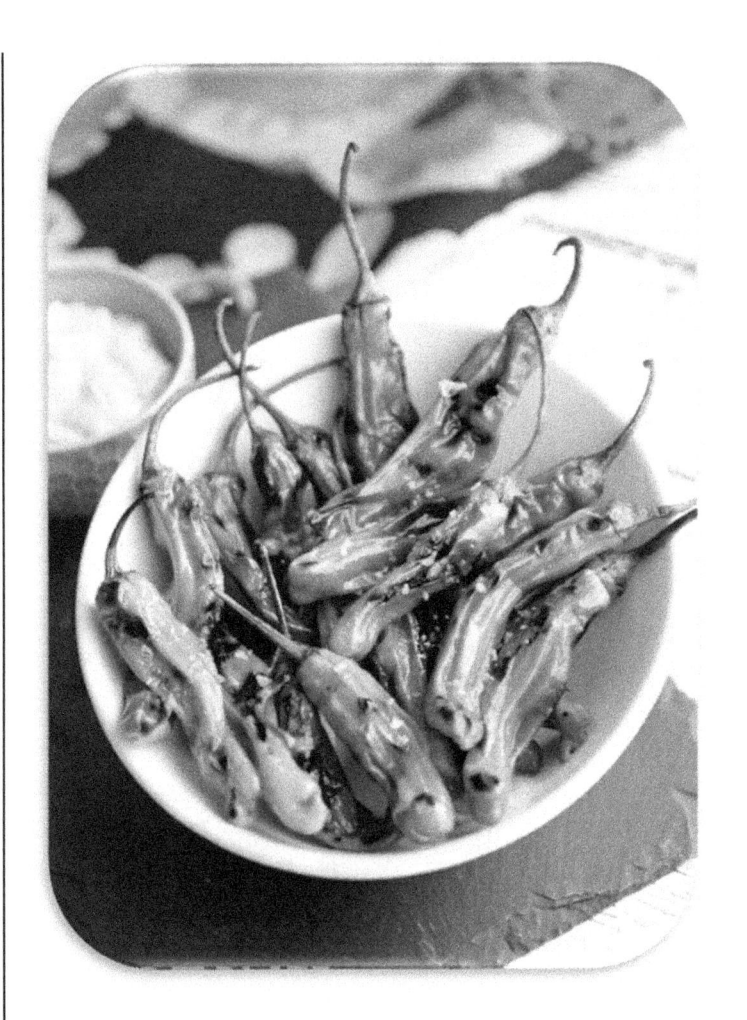

Instructions:

1. Wash the shishito peppers and dry them well.
2. Prepare the paprika mayonnaise: Place the mayonnaise, lemon zest, tomato paste, and paprika in a small bowl, and stir well to combine.
3. Line a baking sheet with paper towels. Heat the oil in a large skillet over high heat, and add the peppers. Cook 2 to 3 minutes, stirring often, until the skins blister. Drain the peppers on the paper towels, and serve immediately with the mayonnaise.

Asparagus with Burrata Cheese and Kale Pesto

Prep time: 20 minutes

Cooking time: 6 minutes

Servings: 4

Nutrients per serving:

Carbohydrates – 4.1 g

Net Carbs – 2 g

Fat – 16.3 g

Protein – 8.8 g

Calories – 174

Ingredients:

- 1 pound asparagus, trimmed
- Olive oil spray
- ½ tsp seasoning salt, divided
- ¼ tsp freshly ground black pepper
- 1 cup kale leaves
- 1 cup packed basil leaves
- 3 Tbsp olive oil
- 2 garlic cloves, minced
- 2 to 3 Tbsp cold water
- 8 ounces burrata cheese

Instructions:

1. Coat the asparagus with olive oil spray. Sprinkle with half the salt and pepper. Heat a skillet, and add the asparagus. Cook for about 6 minutes. Transfer to a platter.
2. Pulse the kale and basil in a food processor seven to eight times. Add the olive oil, garlic, remaining salt, and water; blend until smooth.
3. Cut the burrata into 6 wedges. Top a asparagus with burrata, including its creamy insides. Drizzle with the kale pesto and serve.

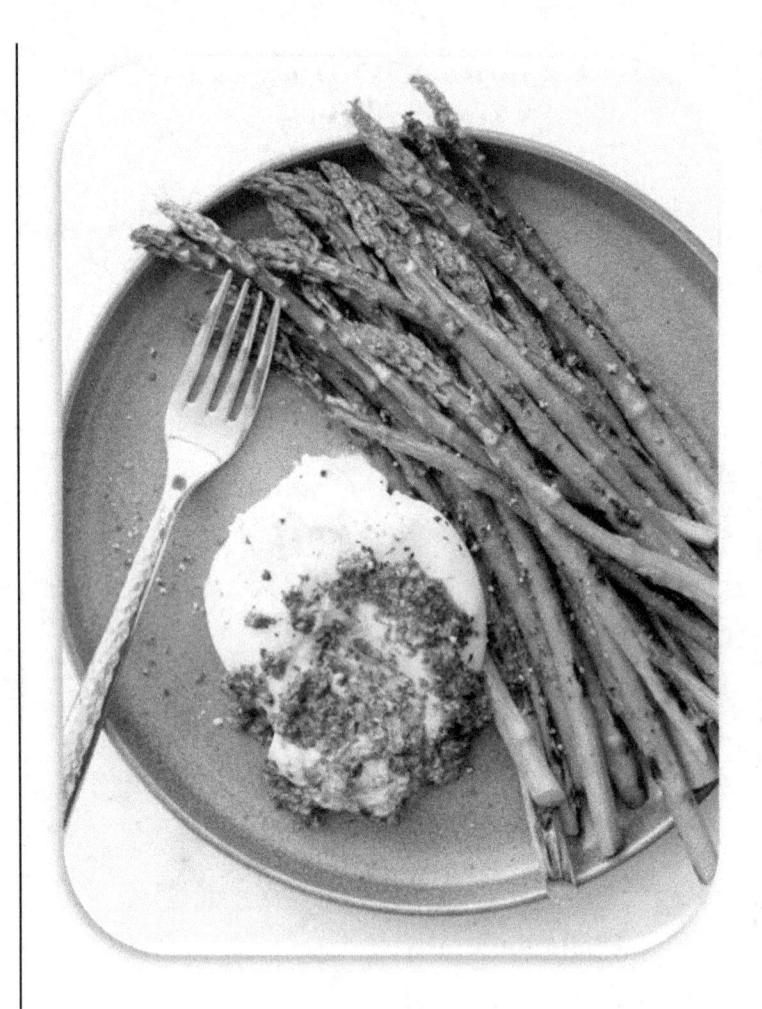

SOUPS AND STEWS

Jalapeño Cheddar Broccoli Soup

Prep time: 10 minutes

Cooking time: 25 minutes

Servings: 4

Nutrients per serving:

Carbohydrates – 13.5 g

Net Carbs – 9.1 g

Fat – 27.4 g

Protein – 18.9 g

Calories – 365

Ingredients:

- 3 Tbsp olive oil
- 1 head broccoli, cut into florets
- 6 jalapeños, seeded and diced
- ½ onion, chopped
- 1 tsp salt
- ½ tsp curry powder or ground turmeric
- ½ tsp freshly ground black pepper
- 2 Tbsp flour
- 1 quart bone broth, or unsalted chicken or beef broth
- ¼ cup heavy cream
- 1 Tbsp hot sauce
- 4 slices (4 ounces) cheddar cheese

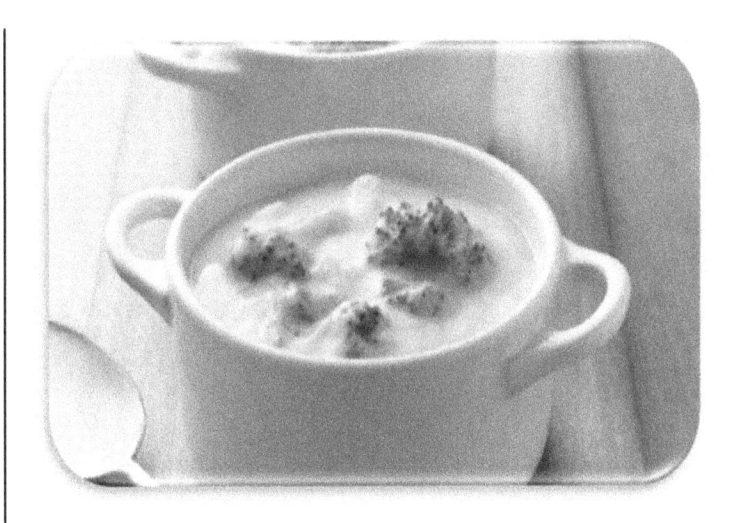

Instructions:

1. Warm the olive oil in a stockpot. Add the broccoli, jalapeños, onion, salt, curry powder or turmeric, and pepper; cook 5 to 6 minutes, stirring often, until the onion begins to brown. Sprinkle with the flour and cook 1 minute more, stirring often, until the flour coats the vegetables. Add the broth and cover.
2. Cook for 15 minutes. Using an immersion blender, blend until smooth. Stir in the heavy cream and hot sauce. Set the oven to broil. Transfer the soup to four oven-safe bowls and top each with one a slice of cheese. Place under the broiler for 3 minutes, until the cheese is melted and bubbly. Serve immediately.

Cauliflower Bisque

Prep time: 15 minutes

Cooking time: 30 minutes

Servings: 4

Nutrients per serving:

Carbohydrates – 8.8 g

Net Carbs – 6.1 g

Fat – 27 g

Protein – 9.3 g

Calories – 339

Ingredients:

- 3 tablespoons unsalted butter
- 1 head cauliflower, cut into florets
- 4 garlic cloves, chopped
- ½ teaspoon salt
- ½ teaspoon freshly grated nutmeg
- ¼ teaspoon freshly ground black pepper
- 1 quart basic bone broth or unsalted chicken or vegetable broth
- 1 tablespoon lemon juice
- ½ cup heavy cream or canned coconut milk
- 4 teaspoons olive oil
- ½ red bell pepper, minced

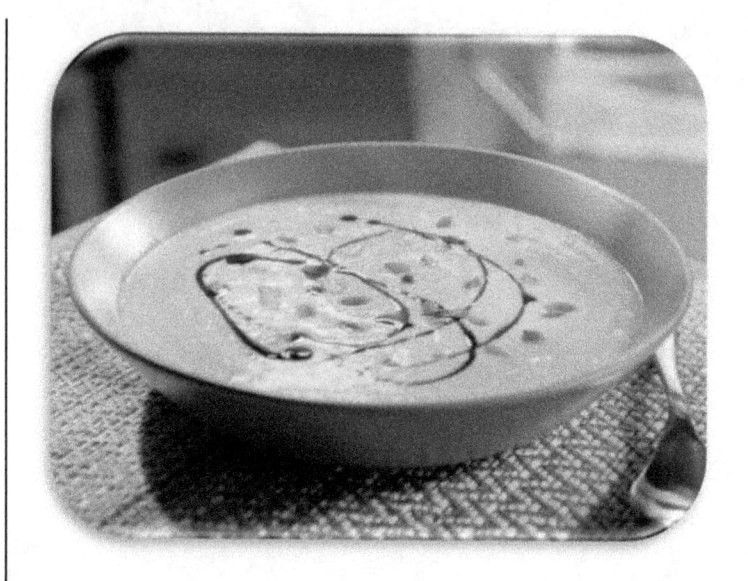

Instructions:

1. Put the butter in a large stockpot, and warm over medium heat, about 1 minute, until the butter foams. Add the cauliflower, garlic, salt, nutmeg, and pepper; cook 5 to 6 minutes, stirring often, until the garlic begins to brown. Add the broth and lemon juice and cover.
2. Cook 15 to 20 minutes, until the cauliflower is fork tender. Using an immersion blender, blend until smooth. Stir in the heavy cream or coconut milk. Spoon into 4 bowls, garnish each serving with the olive oil and bell pepper, and serve immediately.

Spicy Korean Soup with Scallions

Prep time: 15 minutes

Cooking time: 2 hours

Servings: 4

Nutrients per serving:

Carbohydrates – 6.4 g

Net Carbs – 4.7 g

Fat – 21.1 g

Protein – 29.7 g

Calories – 322

Ingredients:

- 1 pound flank steak
- ½ tsp freshly ground black pepper
- 3 Tbsp sesame oil
- 10 ounces mushrooms, such as button, shiitake, or cremini
- 8 scallions, thinly sliced
- 4 garlic cloves, minced
- 2 tsp crushed red pepper flakes
- ¼ tsp salt
- 2 Tbsp soy sauce or tamari
- 2 Tbsp apple cider vinegar
- 1 quart beef broth

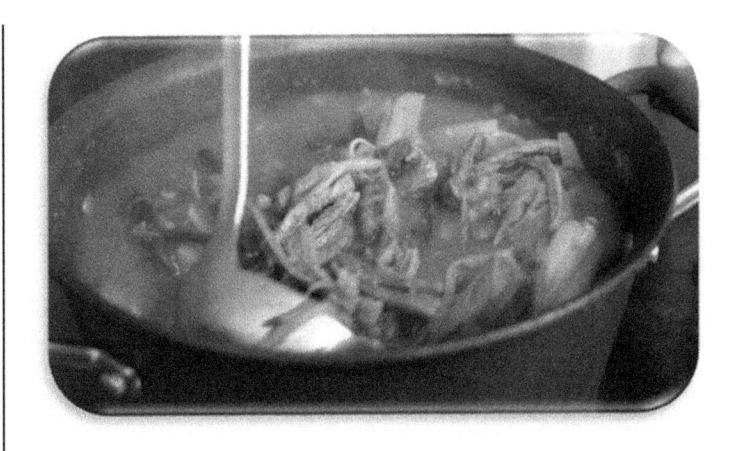

Instructions:

1. Place the flank steak in a large stockpot, and cover with water. Add the black pepper and bring to a boil over high heat. Reduce the heat to low and simmer, covered, for 2 hours, until the meat is very tender. Drain, discarding the liquid, and let the beef cool. Use a fork to shred the meat. Wash and dry the stockpot.
2. Warm the oil in the stockpot over medium-low heat. Add the mushrooms, scallions, garlic, red pepper flakes, and salt, and cook for about 3 minutes, stirring often, until fragrant. Add the shredded beef, soy sauce or tamari, vinegar, and broth. Bring to a simmer and cook for 5 minutes, until the mushrooms are tender. Serve immediately.

Salsa Verde Chicken Soup

Prep time: 10 minutes

Cooking time: 45 minutes

Servings: 4

Nutrients per serving:

Carbohydrates – 8.6 g

Net Carbs – 6.7 g

Fat – 18.3 g

Protein – 33.5 g

Calories – 340

Ingredients:

- 4 chicken breasts, on the bone, skin intact (about 1½ pounds)
- ½ tsp salt
- ½ tsp mild chili powder
- ¼ tsp freshly ground black pepper
- 2 Tbsp olive oil
- ½ red or white onion, minced
- 2 cups cauliflower florets
- 2 cups fresh cilantro leaves and stems, chopped and divided
- 4 garlic cloves
- 1 quart unsalted chicken broth
- ½ cup commercial salsa verde
- ¼ cup sour cream

Instructions:

1. Sprinkle the chicken with the salt, chili powder, and pepper. Warm the oil in a stockpot over medium heat. Add the chicken and cook for 8 minutes, turning a few times, until the chicken is well browned. Transfer the chicken to a plate. Add the onion, cauliflower, half the cilantro, and the garlic, cooking 5 to 6 minutes more, until the vegetables soften.
2. Return the chicken to the stockpot, and cover with the broth. Bring to a simmer and cook 20 to 25 minutes, until the chicken is cooked through. Remove the skin and bones. Shred the chicken. Return it to the soup, and top with the salsa verde and the remaining cilantro. Serve with the sour cream.

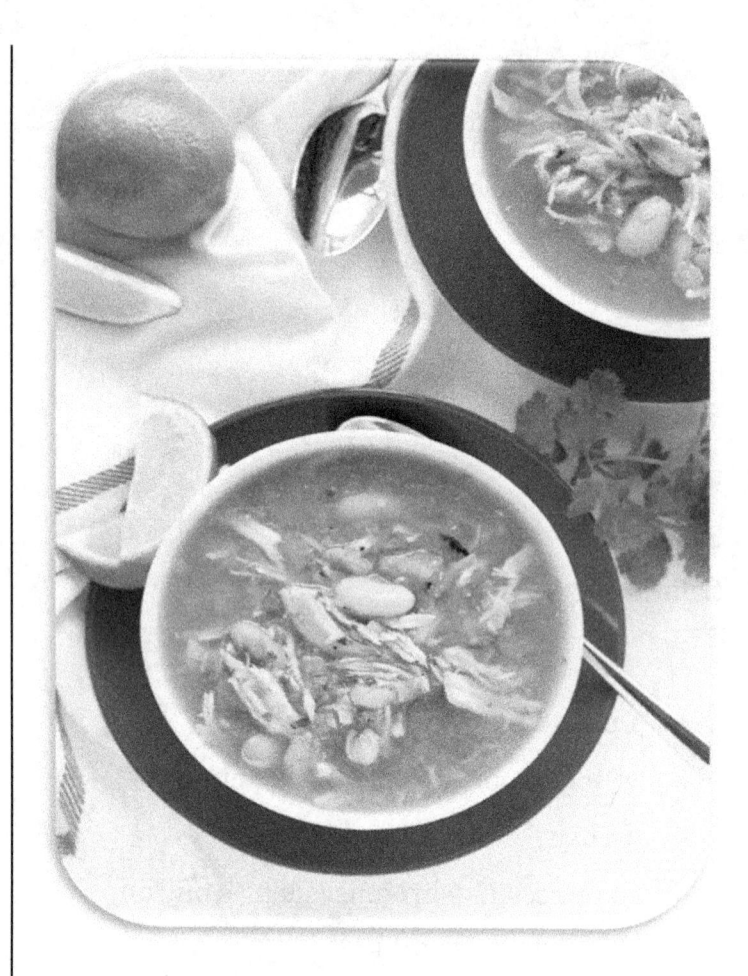

Chicken Vegetable Soup

Prep time: 15 minutes

Cooking time: 1 hour 20 minutes

Servings: 3

Nutrients per serving:

Carbohydrates – 6 g

Net Carbs – 5.5 g

Fat – 12.8 g

Protein – 33.2 g

Calories – 189

Ingredients:

- 1 pound skinless chicken breasts
- ½ cup chopped carrots
- ¼ cup chopped celery
- ¼ cup chopped onion
- Salt and pepper

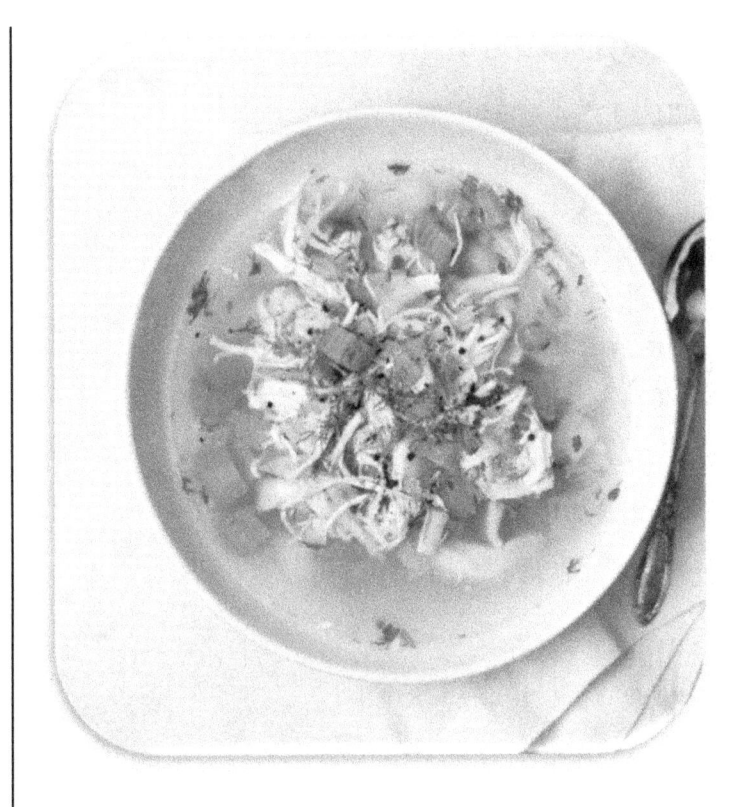

Instructions:

1. Cook chicken breasts in a pot with 2½ cups of water over medium heat for 20 minutes.
2. Remove the chicken from the broth and cut into strips.
3. Put the chicken strips back into the pot with the broth.
4. Season with salt and pepper.
5. Add the rest of the ingredients.
6. Cook for about 1 hour more or until vegetables are done.

Thai Coconut-Shrimp Soup

Prep time: 20 minutes

Cooking time: 10 minutes

Servings: 6

Nutrients per serving:

Carbohydrates – 7 g

Net Carbs – 6 g

Fat – 17 g

Protein – 20 g

Calories – 260

Ingredients:

- 3 cups chicken broth
- 1 (13½-ounce) can unsweetened coconut milk
- 1 (1-inch) piece fresh ginger, peeled, cut into ⅛-inch slices
- 2 Tbsp fish sauce (nam pla or nuoc nam)
- 1 jalapeño, finely chopped
- 1 Tbsp freshly grated lime zest
- 1 tsp granular sugar substitute
- 1 pound medium shrimp, peeled and deveined
- 4 ounces button mushrooms, cut into ¼-inch slices (optional)
- 2 scallions, thinly sliced
- ¼ cup chopped fresh cilantro
- 1 Tbsp fresh lime juice

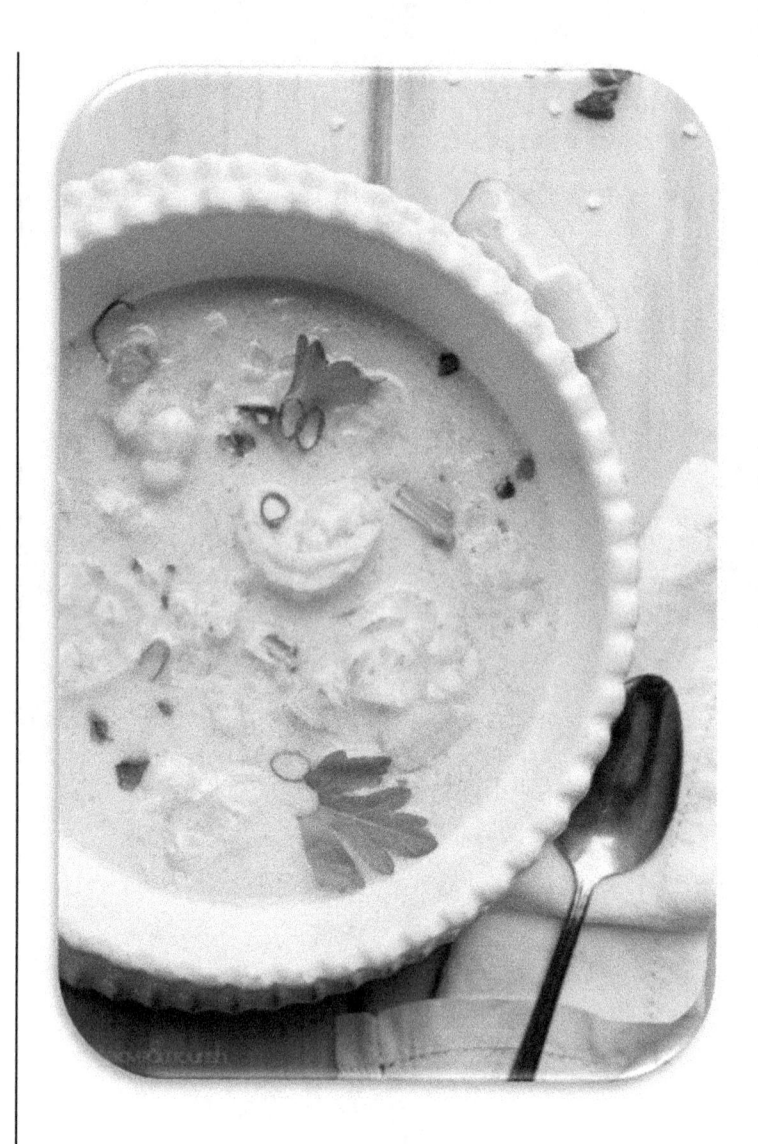

Instructions:

1. Combine first seven ingredients in a soup pot over medium-low heat. Bring to a low boil and simmer for 10 minutes.
2. Add shrimp and mushrooms, if using; simmer until shrimp are cooked through, 3 to 5 minutes. Remove and discard ginger. Stir in the remaining 3 ingredients and serve.

Chinese Hot-and-Sour Soup

Prep time: 10 minutes

Cooking time: 12 minutes

Servings: 4

Nutrients per serving:

Carbohydrates – 5 g

Net Carbs – 3 g

Fat – 7 g

Protein – 9 g

Calories – 110

Ingredients:

- ⅓ cup unseasoned, unsweetened rice vinegar
- 1 Tbsp Dixie Carb Counters Thick-It-Up low-carb thickener
- 1 tsp canola oil
- 1 clove garlic, finely chopped
- ½ cup button mushrooms, thinly sliced
- 4 cups chicken broth
- 1 (10½-ounce) package firm tofu, cut into ¼-inch dice
- 2 Tbsp tamari
- ½ tsp red pepper flakes
- 1 tsp dark (toasted) sesame oil

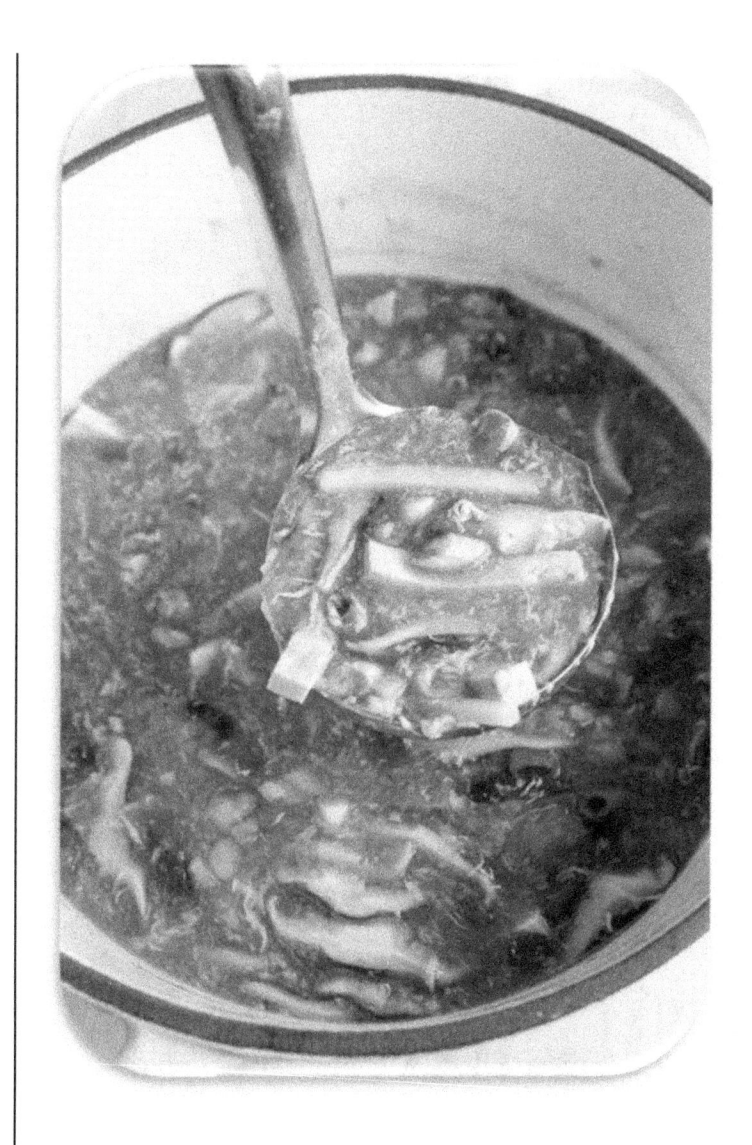

Instructions:

1. Whisk together vinegar and thickener in a small bowl; set aside.
2. Heat canola oil in a soup pot over medium-high heat. Add garlic and sauté until fragrant, about 30 seconds. Add mushrooms and sauté until slightly soft, about 3 minutes.
3. Add broth, tofu, tamari, and pepper flakes; cover and simmer until flavors blend, 5 to 7 minutes. Stir in vinegar mixture and simmer until soup thickens, about 1 minute. Add sesame oil just before serving.

Creamy Cheddar Cheese Soup

Prep time: 10 minutes

Cooking time: 12 minutes

Servings: 4

Nutrients per serving:

Carbohydrates – 9 g

Net Carbs – 7 g

Fat – 32 g

Protein – 17 g

Calories – 390

Ingredients:

- 1 Tbsp butter
- 1 shallot, minced
- 2½ cups vegetable broth
- 1 Tbsp Dixie Carb Counters Thick-It-Up low-carb thickener
- 1½ cups half-and-half
- 8 ounces Cheddar cheese, shredded (2 cups)
- 2 tsp hot paprika
- ½ tsp salt

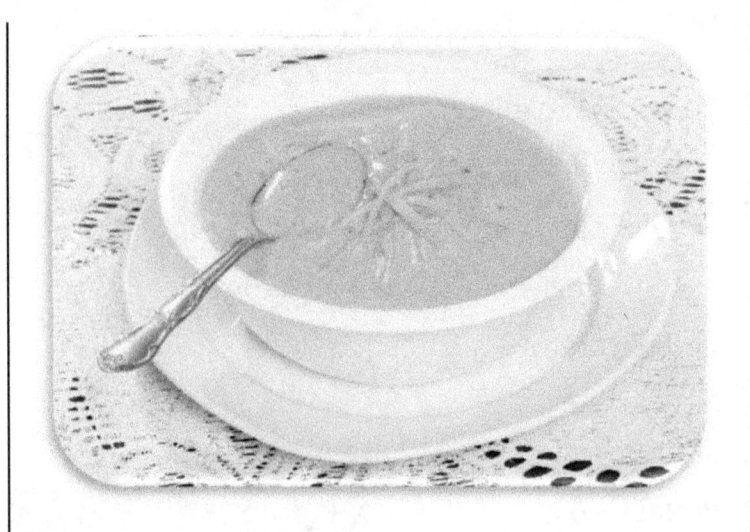

Instructions:

1. Melt butter in a saucepan. Add shallot and sauté until soft, about 3 minutes. Add broth and bring to a simmer. Whisk in thickener; cook until mixture thickens, about 2 minutes.
2. Add half-and-half and simmer, stirring occasionally, until hot. Slowly whisk in cheese until melted and thoroughly combined. Stir in paprika and salt and serve.

Cream of Broccoli Soup

Prep time: 15 minutes

Cooking time: 20 minutes

Servings: 6

Nutrients per serving:

Carbohydrates – 7 g

Net Carbs – 3 g

Fat – 17 g

Protein – 3 g

Calories – 180

Ingredients:

- 4 cups vegetable or chicken broth
- 1 tsp salt
- ¼ tsp freshly ground black pepper
- 1 pound broccoli, cut into florets; stems peeled and cut into 1-inch pieces
- 1 Tbsp Dixie Carb Counters Thick-It-Up low-carb thickener
- 1 cup heavy cream

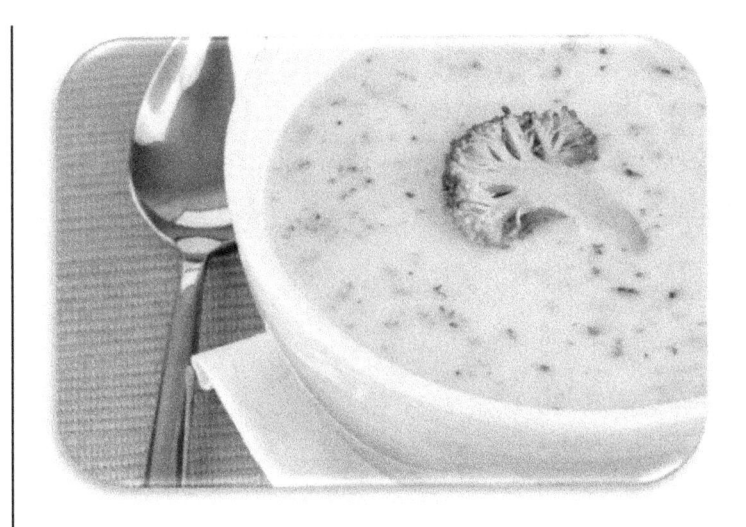

Instructions:

1. Combine broth, salt, and pepper in a soup pot over medium-high heat; bring to a boil. Add broccoli, reduce the heat to medium-low, and simmer until tender, about 15 minutes.
2. Transfer soup to a blender. Blend at low speed to purée. Return soup to the pot; bring back to a simmer over medium-high heat. Whisk in thickener and cream; simmer, whisking occasionally, until thick and hot, about 5 minutes.
3. Serve hot or refrigerate in an airtight container for up to 3 days. Reheat before serving.

Cold Roasted Tomato Soup

Prep time: 15 minutes

Cooking time: 1 hour 45 minutes

Servings: 6

Nutrients per serving:

Carbohydrates – 12 g

Net Carbs – 9 g

Fat – 8 g

Protein – 5 g

Calories – 140

Ingredients:

- 3 pounds fresh plum tomatoes, halved lengthwise
- 1 small yellow onion, peeled and quartered
- 3 Tbsp extra-virgin olive oil
- 3 cloves garlic, peeled
- 1½ tsp salt
- ½ tsp freshly ground black pepper
- 4 cups chicken broth
- 6 Tbsp thinly sliced fresh basil

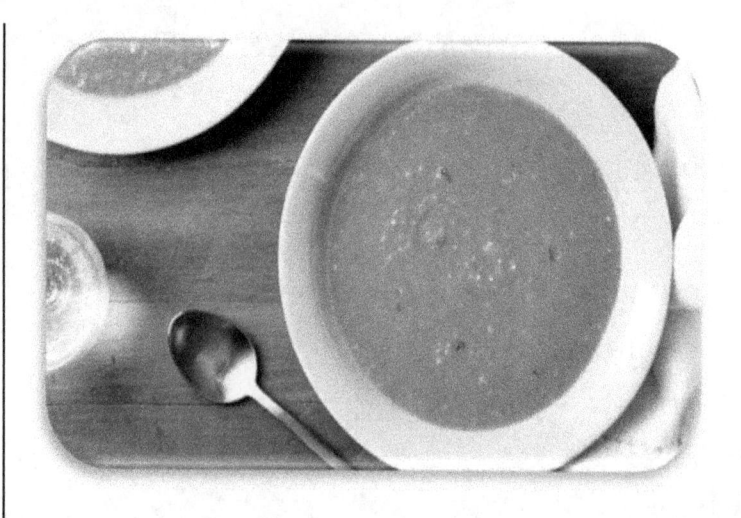

Instructions:

1. Heat oven to 450°F. Line a jelly-roll pan with parchment paper or foil.
2. Combine tomatoes, onion, oil, garlic, salt, and pepper in a mixing bowl; toss to coat. Transfer ingredients to the pan, making sure to include all of the liquid and arranging tomatoes cut side down in a single layer.
3. Roast until tomato skins are puckered and browned, about 20 minutes, rotating pan once halfway through. Let cool.
4. Add garlic and roasted vegetables and any juices to a blender. Holding down blender lid firmly with a folded kitchen towel, blend at low speed until slightly chunky (you may have to work in batches). Add broth and pulse once to combine.
5. Refrigerate until ready to serve or at least 1 hour. Serve, topped with basil.

SALADS

Athenian Salad

Prep time: 15 minutes

Cooking time: none

Servings: 4

Nutrients per serving:

Carbohydrates – 12 g

Net Carbs – 9 g

Fat – 8 g

Protein –14 g

Calories – 280

Ingredients:

- 6 Tbsp extra-virgin olive oil
- 1 clove garlic, finely minced
- 1½ tsp dried oregano, crumbled, or 1 Tbsp fresh oregano, chopped
- ½ tsp salt
- ¼ tsp freshly ground black pepper
- 2 Tbsp + 1 tsp freshly squeezed lemon juice
- ½ small red onion, thinly sliced
- 1½ medium cucumbers, peeled, halved lengthwise, seeded, and thinly sliced
- 1 medium green bell pepper, stemmed, ribs removed, and thinly sliced
- ½ cup pitted quartered kalamata or other black olives
- 12 cherry tomatoes, quartered
- ½ cup crumbled feta cheese

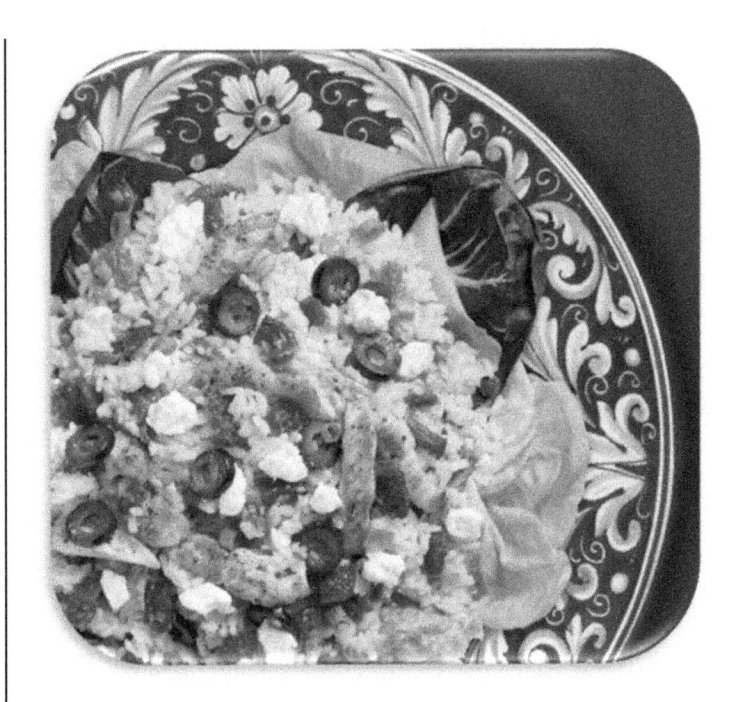

Instructions:

1. Whisk together oil, garlic, oregano, salt and pepper in a small bowl; whisk in lemon juice.
2. Put onion, cucumbers, bell pepper, and olives in a bowl and toss with the dressing. Arrange on a large platter or four individual plates, top with tomatoes and cheese, and serve.

Caprese Salad

Prep time: 15 minutes

Cooking time: none

Servings: 4

Nutrients per serving:

Carbohydrates – 6 g

Net Carbs – 5 g

Fat – 42 g

Protein – 24 g

Calories – 500

Ingredients:

- 1 pound fresh mozzarella, cut into ¼-inch slices
- 4 medium tomatoes, cored and cut into ¼-inch slices
- ¼ cup extra-virgin olive oil
- 4 tsp red wine vinegar
- 1 tsp granular sugar substitute
- ½ tsp salt
- ¼ tsp freshly ground black pepper
- 6 basil leaves, cut into thin strips

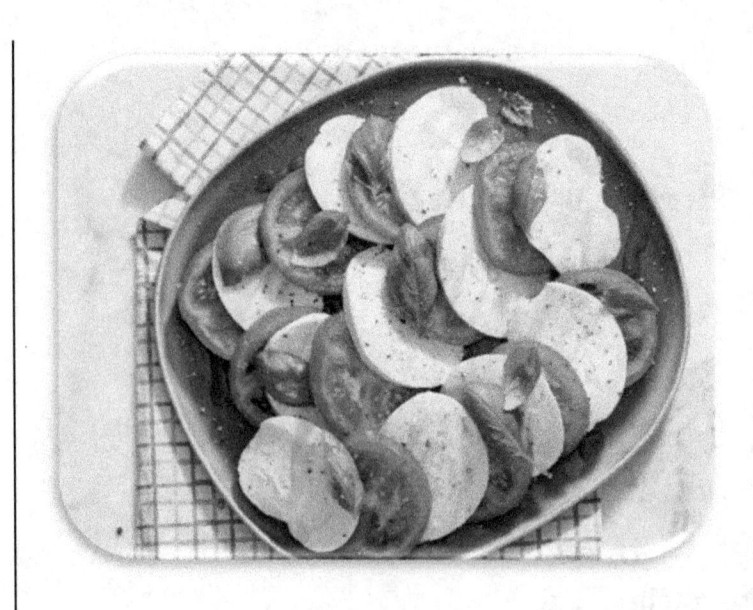

Instructions:

1. Arrange mozzarella and tomatoes on a platter, alternating and overlapping the slices decoratively. Whisk together oil, vinegar, sugar substitute, salt, and pepper in a small bowl. Drizzle over cheese and tomatoes, and then scatter basil on top.

Old Bay Shrimp Salad

Prep time: 15 minutes

Cooking time: 15 minutes

Servings: 4

Nutrients per serving:

Carbohydrates – 4.7 g

Net Carbs – 3 g

Fat – 32.2 g

Protein – 24.4 g

Calories – 409

Ingredients:

- 1 pound frozen cooked small shrimp, defrosted
- 1 cup cauliflower florets, chopped
- 2 celery stalks, thinly sliced
- ¾ cup mayonnaise
- 2 scallions, thinly sliced
- 1 Tbsp Old Bay seasoning or seasoning salt
- 1 head Bibb lettuce, broken into 12 leaves

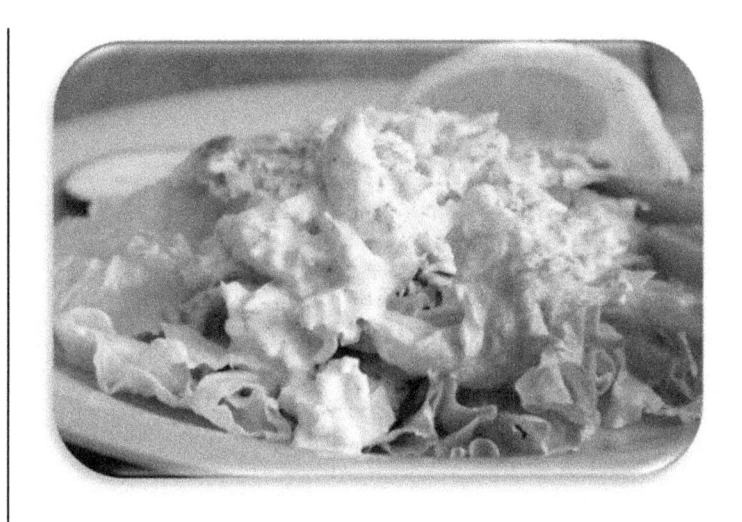

Instructions:

1. Drain the shrimp on paper towels or a kitchen towel to be sure they are dry. Transfer to a bowl along with the cauliflower, celery, mayonnaise, scallions, and Old Bay. Stir well. Set the leaves out on salad plates and divide the salad among the 12 leaves and serve immediately.

Watercress Bacon Salad with Ranch Dressing

Prep time: 15 minutes

Cooking time: none

Servings: 4

Nutrients per serving:

Carbohydrates – 9.6 g

Net Carbs – 4.4 g

Fat – 33.2 g

Protein – 7.5 g

Calories – 353

Ingredients:

- ½ pound watercress
- ½ pound baby spinach
- 2 tomatoes, chopped
- 1 ripe Hass avocado, diced
- 4 slices cooked bacon, crumbled

Ranch Dressing

- ½ cup mayonnaise
- 2 Tbsp canned coconut milk or heavy cream
- 1 tsp apple cider vinegar
- ½ tsp onion powder
- ½ tsp garlic salt
- 1 Tbsp chopped fresh dill or flat-leaf parsley
- ¼ tsp freshly ground black pepper

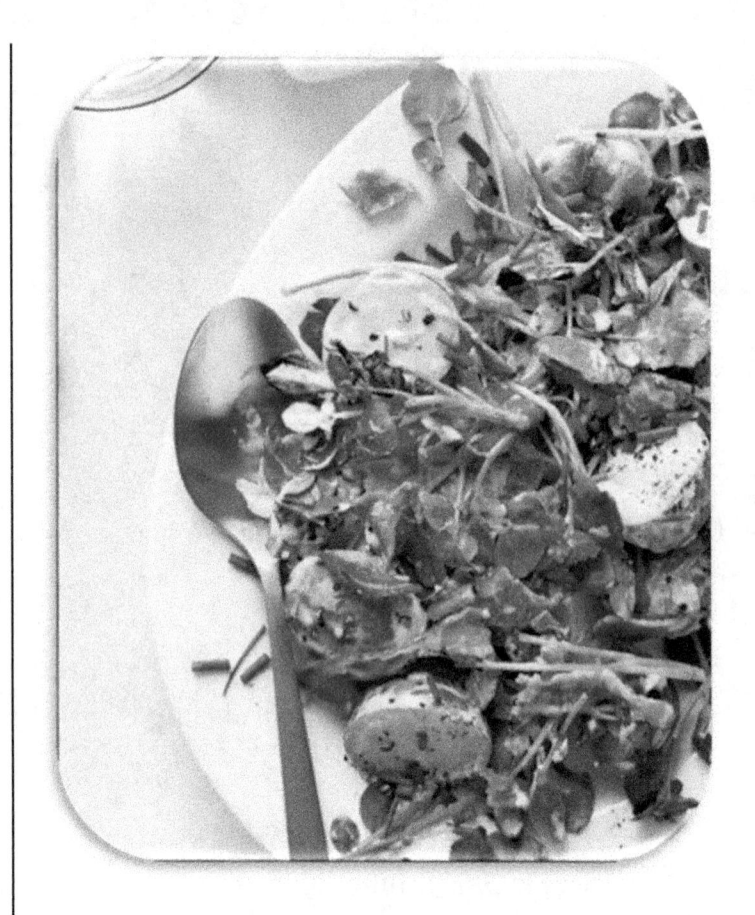

Instructions:

1. Combine the watercress and spinach, tossing well. Put equally on four plates and top with the tomatoes, avocado, and bacon.
2. Place the mayonnaise, coconut milk or heavy cream, vinegar, onion powder, garlic salt, dill or parsley, and black pepper in a large bowl. Whisk well to combine. Serve over the salad.

Shaved Fennel Salad with Lemon Dressing

Prep time: 15 minutes

Cooking time: 4 minutes

Servings: 6

Nutrients per serving:

Carbohydrates – 8 g

Net Carbs – 5 g

Fat – 10 g

Protein – 1 g

Calories – 120

Ingredients:

- ¼ pound green beans, cut into 1½-inch pieces
- ¼ cup extra-virgin olive oil
- 3 Tbsp freshly squeezed lemon juice
- 1 tsp freshly grated lemon zest
- 1 tsp red wine vinegar
- ½ tsp salt
- ½ tsp freshly ground black pepper
- ¼ tsp granular sugar substitute
- 2 medium fennel bulbs, cored, quartered lengthwise, and thinly sliced crosswise
- 2 Tbsp chopped fresh basil

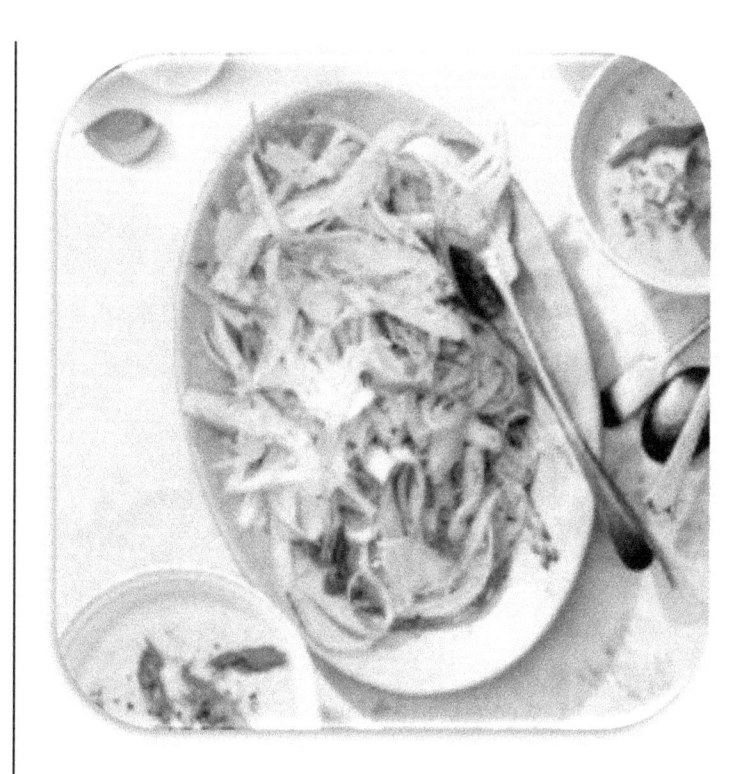

Instructions:

1. In a pot, bBring well-salted water to a boil over high heat. Add green beans and cook for about 4 minutes. Drain; set aside.
2. Combine oil, lemon juice, lemon zest, vinegar, salt, pepper, and sugar substitute in a salad bowl. Add green beans, fennel, and basil and combine; cover and refrigerate at least 30 minutes but no more than 3 hours to let flavors blend. Stir gently before serving.

Cucumber-Dill Salad

Prep time: 15 minutes

Cooking time: none

Servings: 4

Nutrients per serving:

Carbohydrates – 5 g

Net Carbs – 4 g

Fat – 0 g

Protein – 1 g

Calories – 25

Ingredients:

- ½ cup white wine vinegar
- ¼ cup chopped fresh dill
- 2 tsp granular sugar substitute
- 1 tsp salt
- 4 medium cucumbers, thinly sliced

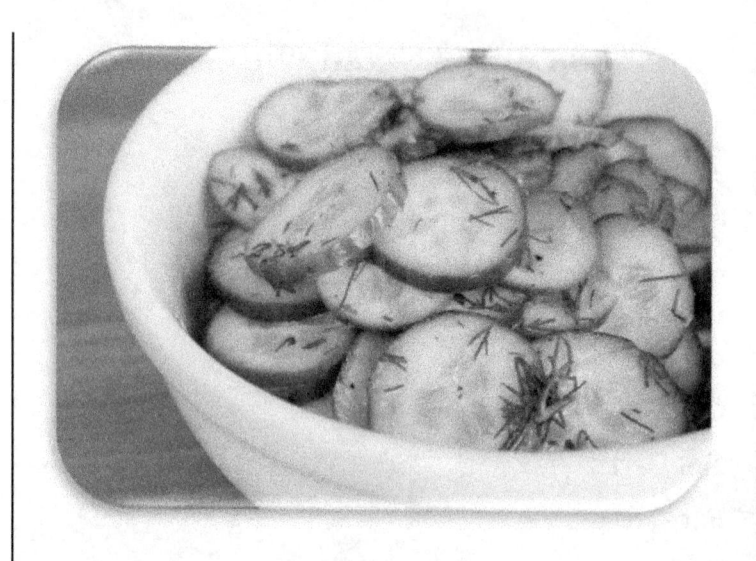

Instructions:

1. Combine vinegar, dill, sugar substitute, and salt in a medium bowl. Add cucumbers and toss gently to coat. Refrigerate 30 minutes to let flavors blend.
2. Drain excess liquid before serving.

Slaw with Vinegar Dressing

Prep time: 20 minutes

Cooking time: none

Servings: 8

Nutrients per serving:

Carbohydrates – 5 g

Net Carbs – 3 g

Fat – 19 g

Protein – 1 g

Calories – 190

Ingredients:

- ⅓ cup white or red wine vinegar
- 1 Tbsp Dijon mustard
- 1 clove garlic, minced
- ⅓ cup extra-virgin olive oil
- ¼ cup chopped fresh parsley
- 4 small scallions, thinly sliced
- ½ tsp salt
- ½ tsp freshly ground black pepper
- ½ large head red or green cabbage, or a combination, shredded (8 cups)

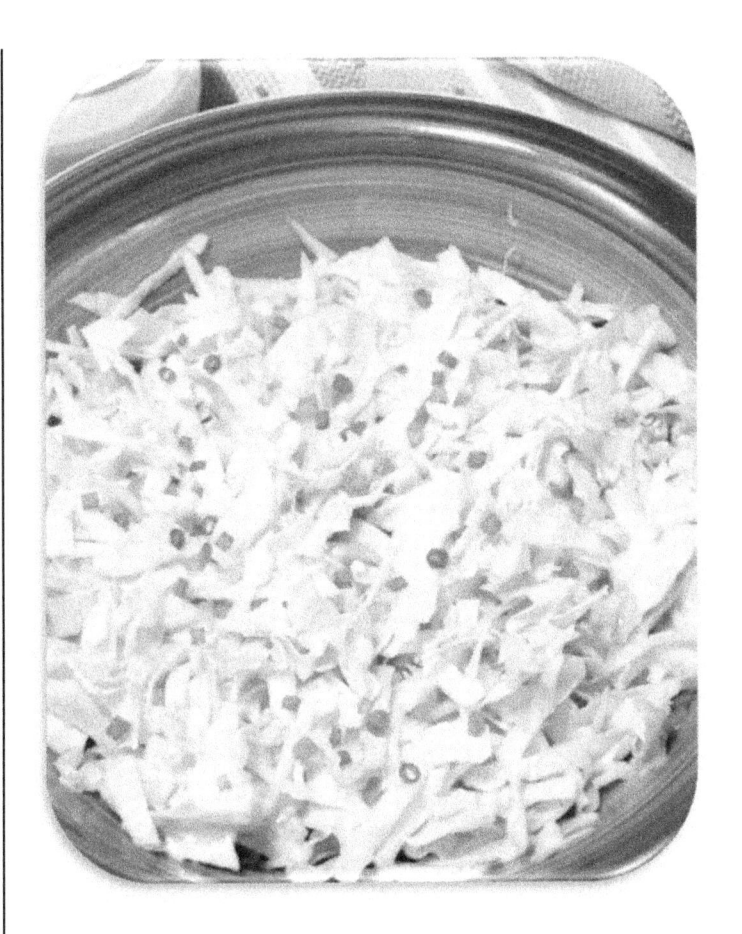

Instructions:

1. Combine vinegar, mustard, and garlic in a salad bowl. Add oil, whisking until dressing thickens. Stir in parsley, scallions, salt, and pepper.
2. Add cabbage; toss to coat. Refrigerate for about 30 minutes before serving.

Wedge Salad with Gorgonzola Dressing

Prep time: 25 minutes

Cooking time: none

Servings: 4

Nutrients per serving:

Carbohydrates – 8.7 g

Net Carbs – 5.2 g

Fat – 27.8 g

Protein – 21.3 g

Calories – 367

Ingredients:

- 4 romaine lettuce hearts
- 4 slices cooked bacon, crumbled
- 1 cup cherry or grape tomatoes, halved
- 2 cup beets, roasted or blanched, chilled, diced or cut into wedges
- 1 cup sliced radishes (or cucumber)

Gorgonzola Dressing

- ½ cup full-fat Greek yogurt
- ½ cup mayonnaise
- ¼ cup Gorgonzola, cut into small pieces
- 2 Tbsp lemon juice
- 1 tsp onion powder
- ½ tsp garlic salt
- ¼ tsp freshly ground black pepper
- ¼ tsp sweet paprika

Instructions:

1. To make the dressing, place the yogurt, mayonnaise, Gorgonzola, lemon juice, onion powder, garlic salt, pepper, and paprika in a medium bowl along with 2 tablespoons warm water and whisk well. Refrigerate until ready to serve.
2. Fill two large bowls with lukewarm water. Add the romaine hearts and soak 3 to 4 minutes while you prepare the dressing. Drain the romaine, wrap in paper towels, and chill in the fridge for at least 1 hour to crisp it up. Cut the romaine hearts in half and place two halves on each plate. Drizzle with the dressing and sprinkle with pepper. Top with the bacon, tomatoes, beets, radishes. Serve with the remaining dressing.

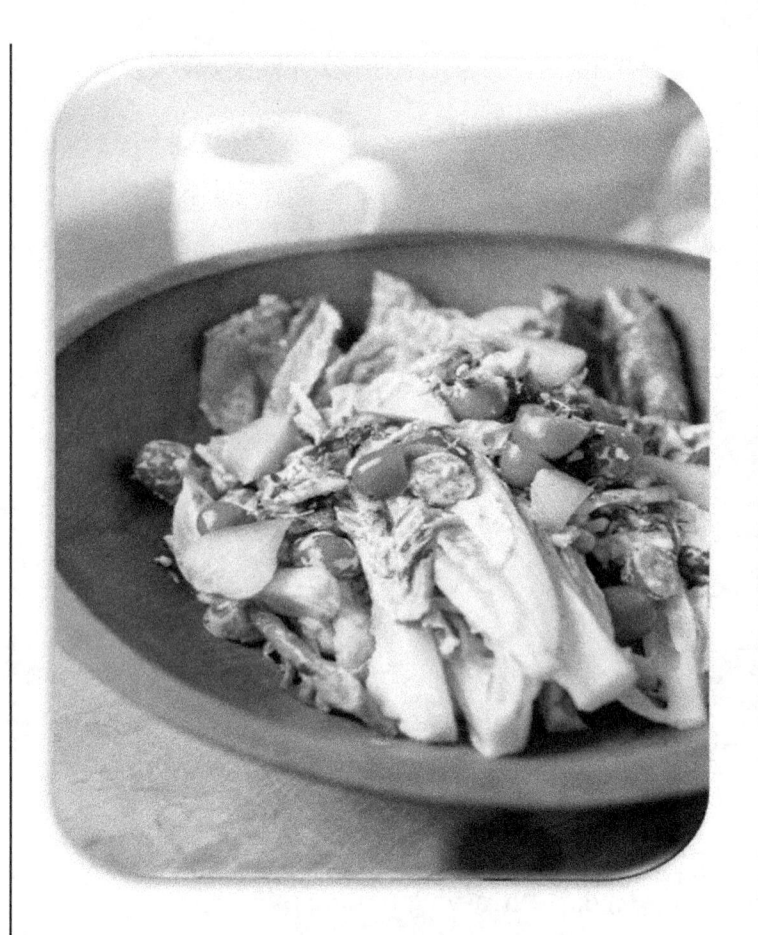

Mixed Power Greens Prosciutto-Wrapped Chicken Tenders

Prep time: 25 minutes

Cooking time: 8 minutes

Servings: 4

Nutrients per serving:

Carbohydrates – 9.3 g

Net Carbs – 4.8 g

Fat – 13.1 g

Protein – 33.5 g

Calories – 295

Ingredients:

- Olive oil spray
- 4 slices prosciutto (about 1 ounce)
- 8 chicken tenders (1 pound)
- 5 ounces mixed "power greens" or baby spinach
- ½ pound green beans, trimmed and chopped

Mustard Vinaigrette

- 3 Tbsp olive oil
- 2 Tbsp red wine or apple cider vinegar
- 1 tsp Dijon mustard
- ½ tsp garlic salt
- ¼ tsp freshly ground black pepper

Instructions:

1. Preheat the oven to 400°F. Coat a baking sheet with olive oil spray.
2. To make the dressing, place the olive oil, vinegar, mustard, salt, and pepper in a small bowl and whisk well.
3. Cut the prosciutto slices in half diagonally, making a total of 8 pieces. Wrap each chicken tender in ½ slice of prosciutto and place on the baking sheet.
4. Coat the tops of the tenders with olive oil spray, and bake 6 to 8 minutes, until the prosciutto is crisped and the chicken is cooked through and no longer pink in the center when sliced.
5. Divide the greens among four plates along with the green beans. Transfer the tenders to the salad, and drizzle with the dressing. Serve immediately.

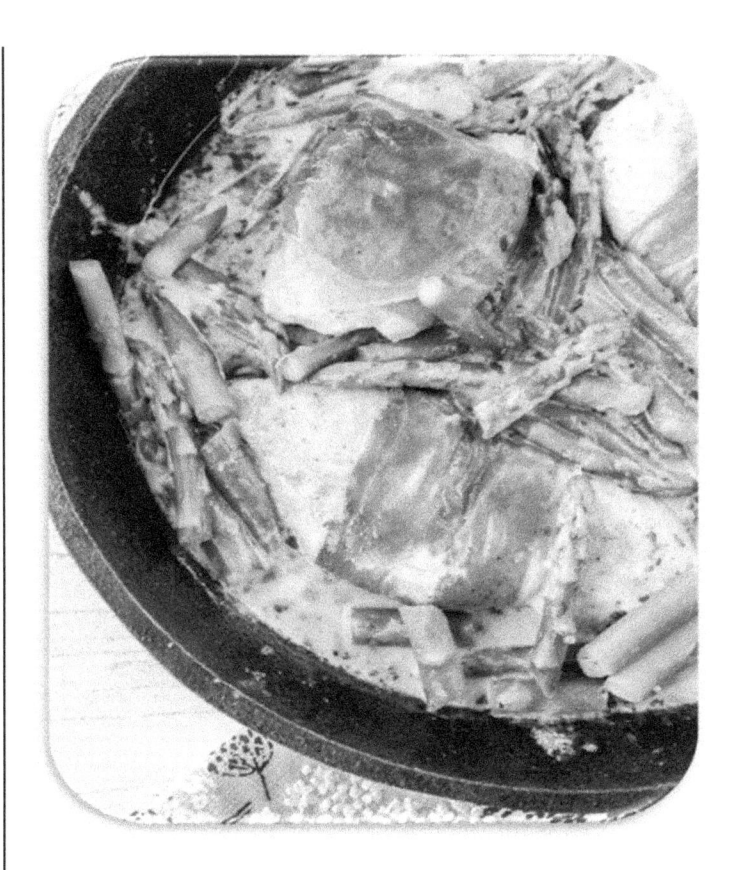

Tomato and Red Onion Salad

Prep time: 20 minutes

Cooking time: none

Servings: 8

Nutrients per serving:

Carbohydrates – 4 g

Net Carbs – 3 g

Fat – 9 g

Protein – 1 g

Calories – 100

Ingredients:

- 3 Tbsp red wine vinegar
- 2 tsp Dijon mustard
- ¾ tsp salt
- ½ tsp freshly ground black pepper
- 5 Tbsp extra-virgin olive oil
- 3 large tomatoes, cut into 1-inch pieces
- ½ small red onion, thinly sliced
- ½ seedless cucumber, cut into ⅓-inch dice
- ¼ cup chopped fresh basil or dill
- 2 Tbsp capers, rinsed and drained

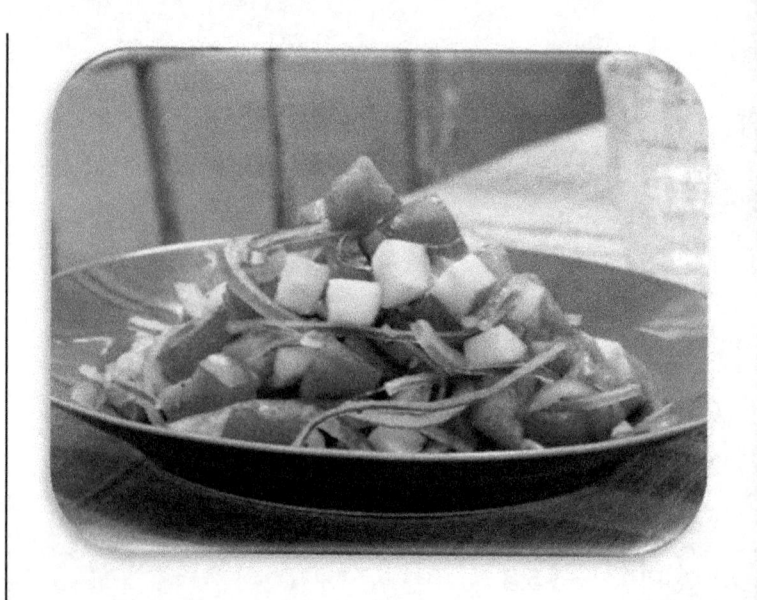

Instructions:

1. Combine first four ingredients in a salad bowl. Add oil, whisking until dressing thickens.
2. Add tomatoes, cucumbers, onion, basil, and capers; toss gently and serve right away.

MAIN DISHES

Mushroom-Herb-Stuffed Chicken Breasts

Prep time: 25 minutes

Cooking time: 40 minutes

Servings: 4

Nutrients per serving:

Carbohydrates – 3 g

Net Carbs – 2 g

Fat – 14 g

Protein – 41 g

Calories – 300

Ingredients:

- 3 Tbsp butter, divided
- ½ pound fresh shiitake mushrooms, wiped clean, trimmed, and minced
- ½ small yellow or white onion, minced
- 2 cloves garlic, minced
- 2 Tbsp dry sherry
- 3 Tbsp chopped fresh parsley
- ½ tsp chopped fresh thyme
- ¾ tsp salt, divided
- ⅛ tsp freshly ground black pepper
- 4 bone-in chicken breast halves (about 2 pounds) with skin

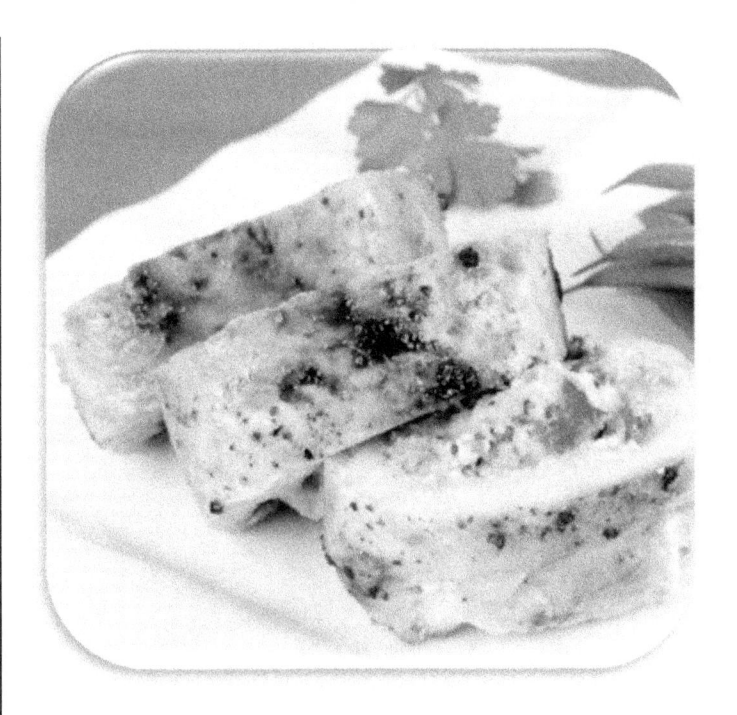

Instructions:

1. Heat oven to 400°F.
2. Melt 2 Tbsp butter in a skillet. Add mushrooms and onion; sauté until mushrooms have released their liquid, about 5 minutes. Stir in garlic and sherry; cook 1 minute longer. Remove from heat; stir in parsley, thyme, ½ tsp salt, and pepper.
3. Using a thin sharp knife, cut a pocket in the thicker part of each breast, stuff mushroom mixture into pockets.
4. Set chicken, skin side up, in a 9-by-13-inch baking pan. Melt remaining tablespoon butter and brush on chicken. Season with remaining ¼ teaspoon salt. Bake until cooked through, about 35 minutes. Serve warm.

Jerk Chicken

Prep time: 25 minutes

Cooking time: 40 minutes

Servings: 4

Nutrients per serving:

Carbohydrates – 7 g

Net Carbs – 5 g

Fat – 17 g

Protein – 34 g

Calories – 320

Ingredients:

- 6 scallions, sliced
- 2 cloves garlic, minced
- 3 Scotch bonnet chili peppers, seeded and minced
- ¼ cup canola oil
- 2 Tbsp freshly squeezed lime juice
- 2 Tbsp ground allspice
- 4 tsp mustard powder
- 2 tsp salt
- 2 tsp granular sugar substitute
- 1 tsp ground cinnamon
- 4 bone-in, skin-on chicken breast halves

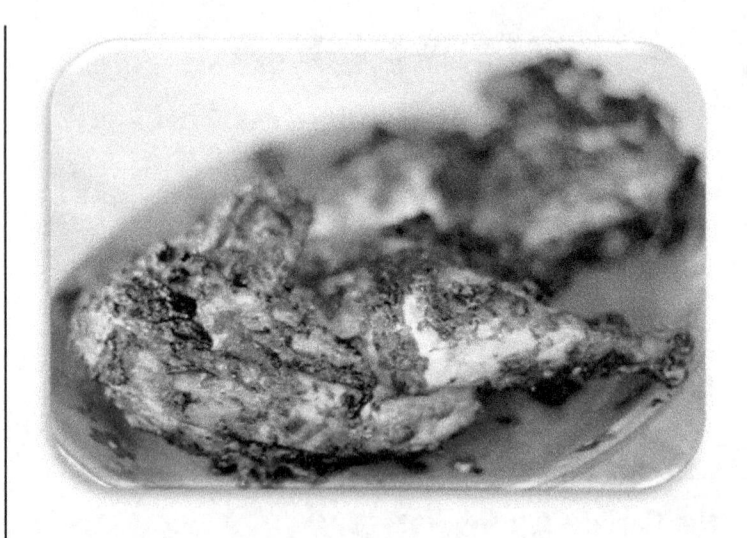

Instructions:

1. Combine all ingredients except the chicken in a food processor or blender; purée. Transfer to a resealable plastic bag or glass baking dish; add chicken and turn to coat. Refrigerate overnight, turning once.
2. Heat oven to 450°F.
3. Line a baking sheet with foil. Remove chicken from marinade, letting excess drain off; transfer to the baking sheet. Bake until just cooked through, 30–40 minutes. Serve.

Roast Beef with Greek Yogurt-Horseradish Sauce

Prep time: 25 minutes

Cooking time: 1 hour 30 minutes

Servings: 14

Nutrients per serving:

Carbohydrates – 1.5 g

Net Carbs – 1.2 g

Fat – 6.3 g

Protein – 37.7 g

Calories – 223

Ingredients:

- 1 tsp garlic salt
- 1 tsp sweet paprika
- 1 tsp freshly ground black pepper
- 1 (5-pound) top or bottom round beef roast

Horseradish Sauce

- 2 Tbsp grated fresh horseradish
- 1 cup full-fat Greek yogurt
- 1 Tbsp lemon juice
- 1 cucumber, peeled, seeded, and grated

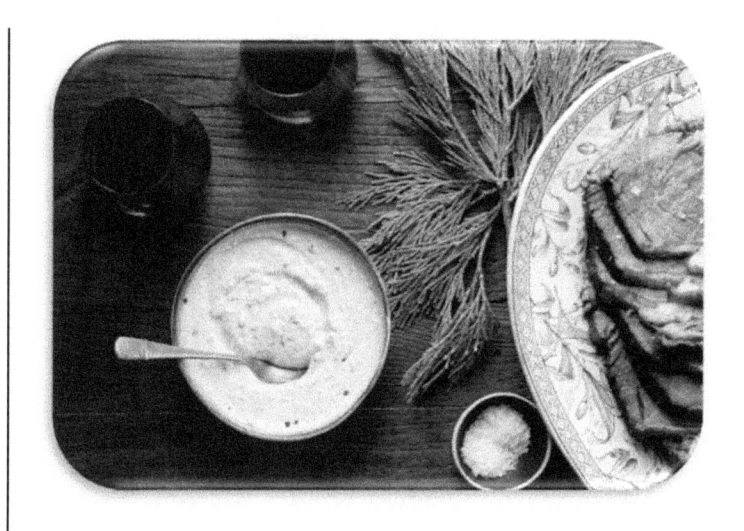

Instructions:

1. Preheat the oven to 375°F.
2. To make the sauce, place the horseradish, yogurt, lemon juice, and cucumber in a medium bowl. Stir well to combine, and refrigerate.
3. Place the garlic salt, paprika, and pepper in a small bowl, and mix well with a spoon. Sprinkle the roast with the spices, and transfer to a 2-quart baking dish.
4. Transfer the roast to the oven, and cook for 1 hour to 1 hour 30 minutes. Set aside for 5 minutes to allow the juices to redistribute.
5. Slice the roast beef, and serve immediately with the Horseradish Sauce.

Chicken-Fried Steak

Prep time: 20 minutes

Cooking time: 6 minutes

Servings: 6

Nutrients per serving:

Carbohydrates – 8 g

Net Carbs – 4 g

Fat – 38 g

Protein – 37 g

Calories – 520

Ingredients:

- 1 cup all purpose baking mix
- 1 tsp garlic powder
- 1 tsp hot paprika
- 1½ tsp salt, divided
- ½ tsp freshly ground black pepper
- 2 large eggs
- ½ cup buttermilk
- ¾ cups canola oil
- 1½ pounds London broil, cut into ¼-inch thick slices and patted dry
- 1 Tbsp fresh chopped parsley
- 1 lemon, cut into wedges

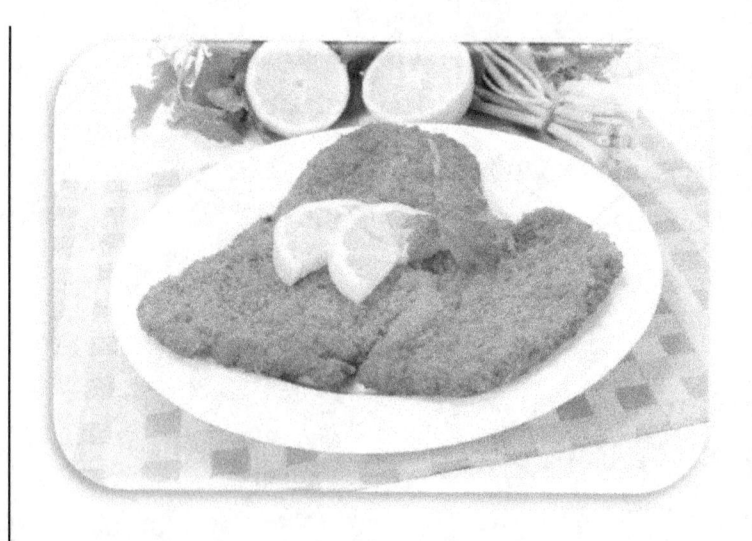

Instructions:

1. Whisk baking mix, garlic powder, paprika, 1 teaspoon salt, and pepper in a shallow bowl. Whisk eggs, buttermilk, and ½ teaspoon salt in another shallow bowl.
2. Heat oil in a large skillet until very hot. Dredge steaks in seasoned baking mix and shake off excess. Dip in egg wash, shake off excess, and dredge again in baking mix. Fry steaks in 2 batches, turning once, about 3 minutes per side.
3. Put on a warm platter and garnish with parsley and lemon wedges.

Slow-Cooked Pork Shoulder

Prep time: 15 minutes

Cooking time: 3 hours

Servings: 8

Nutrients per serving:

Carbohydrates – 1 g

Net Carbs – 1 g

Fat – 30 g

Protein – 43 g

Calories – 460

Ingredients:

- 1 boneless shoulder (butt) pork roast, about 4 pounds
- ½ cup beef broth
- 2 Tbsp tamari
- ½ tsp hot pepper sauce
- 2 Tbsp red wine or cider vinegar
- 2 Tbsp sugar-free pancake syrup
- 1 tsp ground cumin

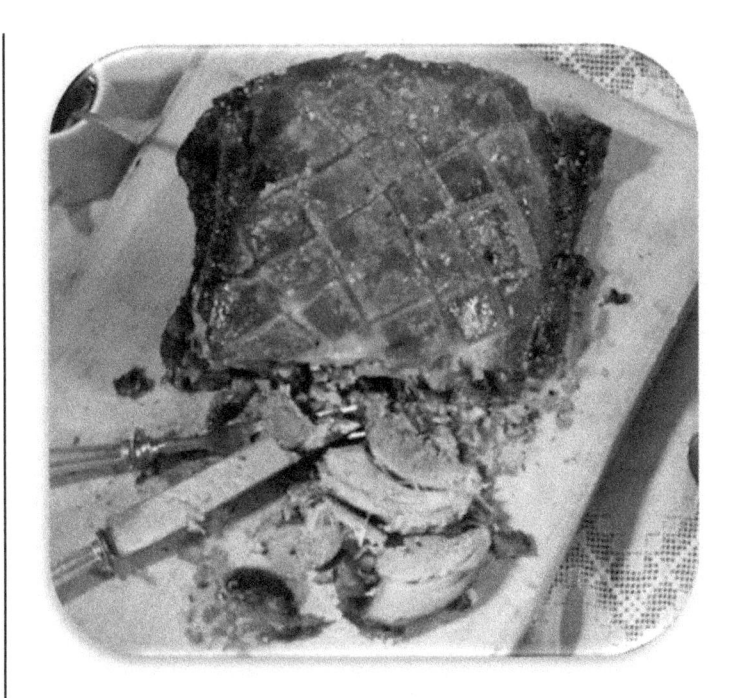

Instructions:

1. Heat oven to 325°F. Set pork in a casserole or Dutch oven with a lid. Combine broth, tamari, hot pepper sauce, vinegar, syrup, and cumin; pour over pork. Cover and bake until fork-tender, about 3 hours.
2. Set aside for about 10 minutes before slicing or shredding, and serve.

Fontina-and-Prosciutto-Stuffed Veal Chops

Prep time: 25 minutes

Cooking time: 10 minutes

Servings: 4

Nutrients per serving:

Carbohydrates – 1 g

Net Carbs – 1 g

Fat – 25 g

Protein – 48 g

Calories – 440

Ingredients:

- 2 ounces fontina cheese, shredded (½ cup)
- 1 ounce prosciutto, chopped
- ¼ cup chopped fresh basil
- 4 (8-ounce) veal rib chops
- ¾ tsp salt
- ½ tsp freshly ground black pepper

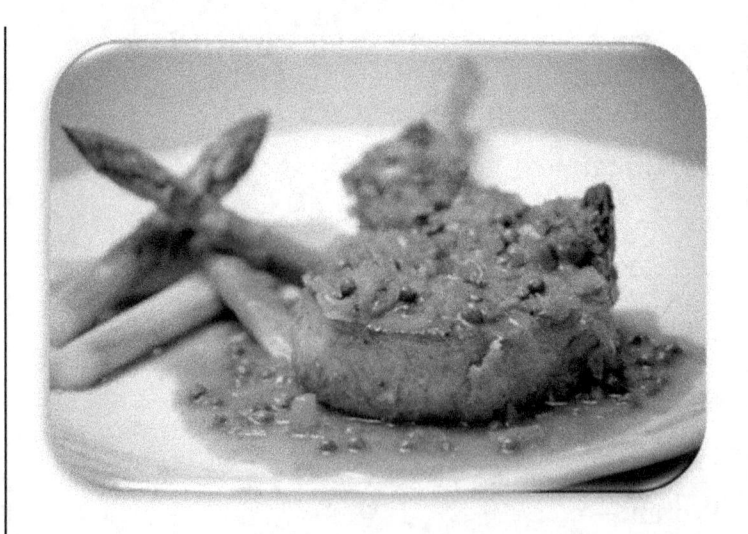

Instructions:

1. Combine cheese, prosciutto, and basil in a small bowl.
2. Cut a horizontal pocket in each chop. Season chops with salt and pepper. Fill with cheese mixture; secure openings with toothpicks.
3. Prepare a medium-high-heat grill or heat a grill pan until very hot. Grill chops until they are browned and just lose their pink color throughout, about 5 minutes per side. Serve hot.

Almond-Crusted Catfish Fingers

Prep time: 15 minutes

Cooking time: 5 minutes

Servings: 4

Nutrients per serving:

Carbohydrates – 11 g

Net Carbs – 6 g

Fat – 58 g

Protein – 39 g

Calories – 720

Ingredients:

- ¾ cup or more canola oil, for frying
- 2 large eggs
- 1 Tbsp cold water
- 1½ Tbsp Old Bay Seasoning or any Cajun spice blend
- ¾ tsp salt
- 1½ pounds catfish fillets, cut into 1½-inch-wide strips
- ¼ cup all purpose baking mix
- 1 cup almond meal
- 1 lemon, cut into wedges

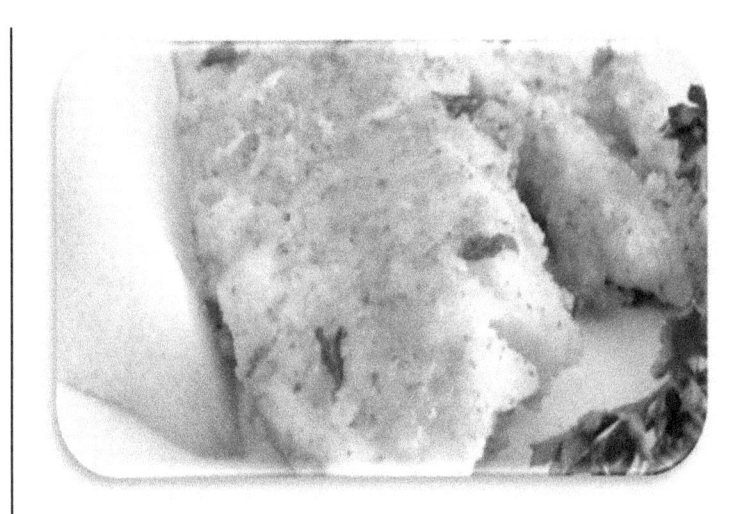

Instructions:

1. Heat oil in a heavy-bottomed saucepan or Dutch oven over high heat until shimmering.
2. Lightly beat eggs in a small bowl; whisk in water and spice blend.
3. Dredge catfish in baking mix and shake off any excess. Dip into egg mixture and then dredge in almond meal. Slip catfish pieces into oil; fry 4 or 5 at a time until golden, about 2 minutes per side. Drain fish on paper towels. Serve hot with lemon wedges.

Baked Bluefish with Garlic and Lime

Prep time: 15 minutes

Cooking time: 12 minutes

Servings: 4

Nutrients per serving:

Carbohydrates – 6 g

Net Carbs – 4 g

Fat – 14 g

Protein – 34 g

Calories – 290

Ingredients:

- 2 Tbsp virgin olive oil, plus more for baking dish
- 2 cloves garlic, minced
- ¼ tsp red pepper flakes
- 1½ pounds bluefish fillets with skin
- Salt, to taste
- 3 limes, quartered

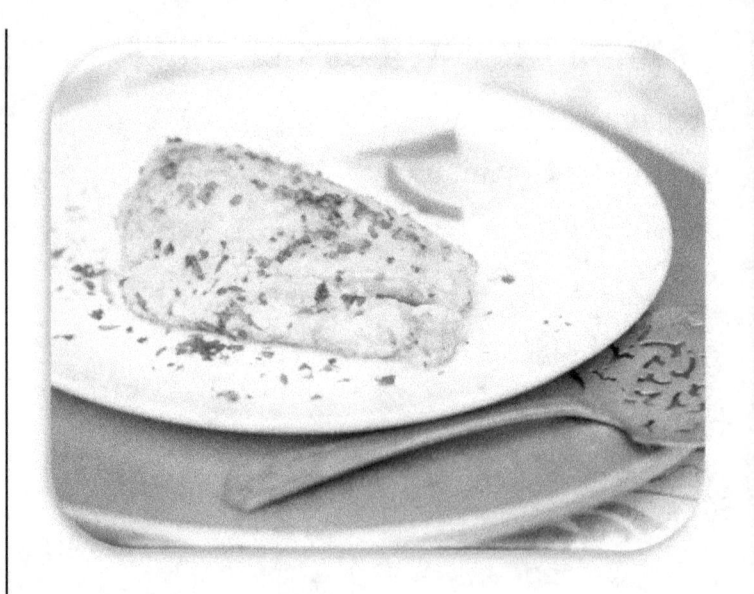

Instructions:

1. Grease a 9-by-13-inch baking dish with oil, and put it in the oven and heat to 425°F.
2. Combine oil, garlic, and red pepper flakes in a small bowl. Rub fillets with garlic mixture and season generously with salt to taste.
3. Using potholders, carefully remove baking dish from oven; add fillets, skin side down, and limes. Bake until fish is opaque and flakes easily, 10–12 minutes. Serve, squeezing limes over fish once they are cool enough to handle.

Baked Salmon with Mustard-Nut Crust

Prep time: 20 minutes

Cooking time: 15 minutes

Servings: 4

Nutrients per serving:

Carbohydrates – 5 g

Net Carbs – 3 g

Fat – 35 g

Protein – 39 g

Calories – 490

Ingredients:

- 4 (6-ounce) center-cut fillets of salmon
- 2 Tbsp coarse-grain Dijon mustard
- ¼ cup fine bread crumbs
- ½ cup finely ground pecans or walnuts
- 1 Tbsp chopped fresh parsley

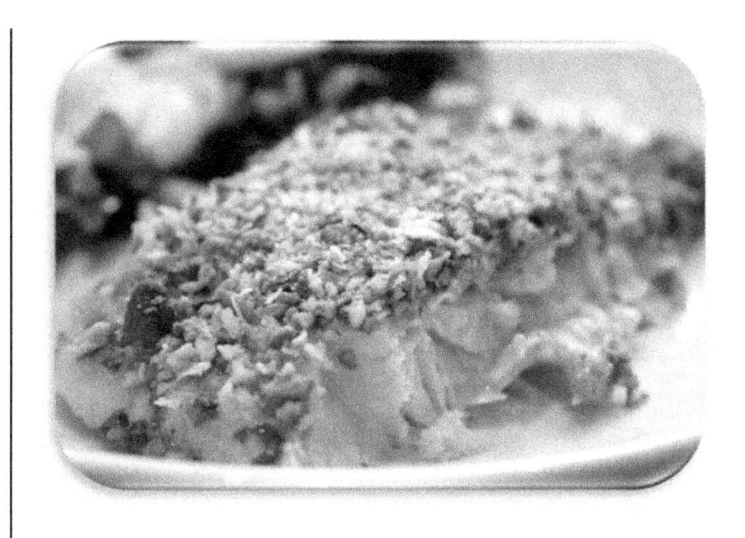

Instructions:

1. Preheat oven to 450°F. Line a baking sheet with foil and place fillets on the sheet. Spread ½ Tbsp mustard on each fillet, covering top evenly.
2. Combine bread crumbs, nuts, and parsley in a small bowl. Divide among fillets, pressing onto mustard to form an even crust. Bake until just cooked through, about 10–15 minutes, being careful not to burn the nuts. Serve right away.

Beef Bourguignon

Prep time: 30 minutes

Cooking time: 3 hours

Servings: 4

Nutrients per serving:

Carbohydrates – 8.9 g

Net Carbs – 7.2 g

Fat – 30.3 g

Protein – 28.2 g

Calories – 461

Ingredients:

- 1 pound beef stew meat
- 1 Tbsp flour mix
- ½ tsp salt
- ¼ tsp freshly ground black pepper
- 2 Tbsp unsalted butter
- 2 Tbsp olive oil
- ¼ pound bacon, chopped
- 10 ounces mushrooms, such as cremini, trimmed and sliced
- ½ onion, chopped
- 4 garlic cloves, minced
- 2 Tbsp tomato paste
- 1 tsp fresh thyme leaves
- 1 cup dry red wine
- 2 cups beef broth

Instructions:

1. Put the beef on a plate, and sprinkle with the flour mix, salt, and pepper. Toss to coat evenly. Set aside.
2. Warm the butter and olive oil in a large stockpot or Dutch oven over medium-high heat. Add the beef and cook 4 to 5 minutes, turning occasionally, until the coating browns. Transfer the beef to a plate.
3. Add in the bacon and cook for 5 minutes, stirring often, scraping up any brown bits that stick to the inside of the pot. Add the mushrooms, onion, and garlic; cook 4 to 5 minutes, stirring often, until the mushrooms soften and the onion is brown. Then reduce the heat to low, and add the tomato paste and thyme, cooking 1 minute more, until the tomato paste is fragrant. Pour in the red wine and broth, and increase the heat to high. Return the beef to the pot, and bring to a boil, then immediately reduce to a simmer and cover. Cook for 3 hours, until the beef is tender and the sauce thickens. Serve immediately.

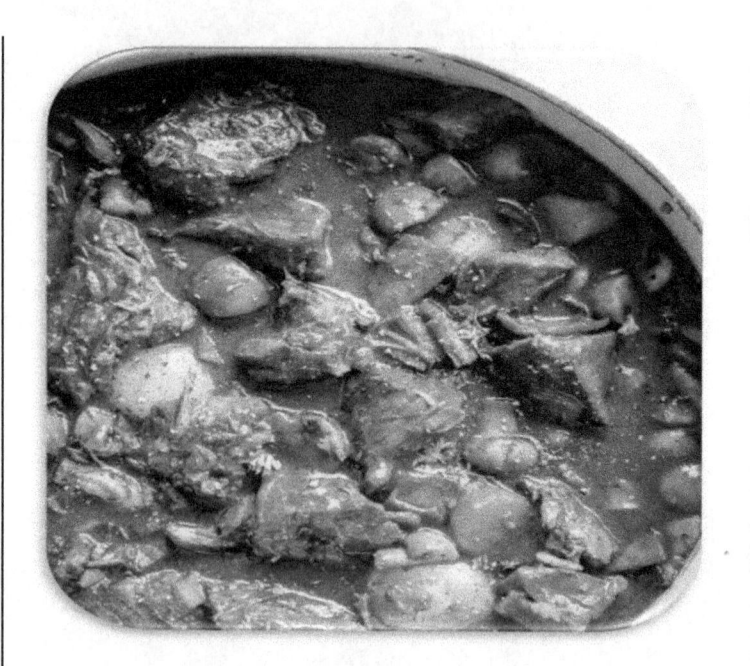

Roasted Fennel and Cod with Moroccan Olives

Prep time: 20 minutes

Cooking time: 40 minutes

Servings: 4

Nutrients per serving:

Carbohydrates – 11.2 g

Net Carbs – 6.4 g

Fat – 18.4 g

Protein – 32.4 g

Calories – 335

Ingredients:

- 2 fennel bulbs, trimmed and thinly sliced
- Zest of 1 lemon, save lemon
- 1 Tbsp olive oil
- ½ tsp garlic salt
- 1½ pounds cod fillets
- ½ cup black Moroccan olives, pitted
- ¼ cup chopped dill or cilantro
- ½ tsp hot paprika or ¼ tsp crushed red pepper flakes
- ¼ tsp salt
- ¼ tsp freshly ground black pepper
- 4 Tbsp unsalted butter

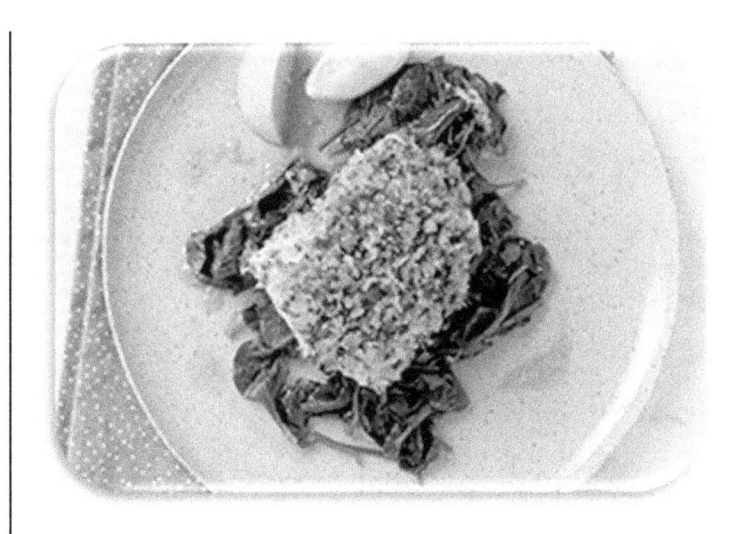

Instructions:

1. Preheat the oven to 400°F. Place the fennel in a 7-by-11-inch baking dish. Scatter the lemon zest over the fennel, and add the olive oil and garlic salt. Toss well. Bake for about 15 minutes, until the edges of the fennel start to brown.
2. Cut the zested lemon into quarters. Place the fish on top of the fennel, as well as the lemon wedges, and sprinkle with the olives, dill or cilantro, paprika or chili flakes, salt, and pepper. Top each piece of fish with 1 tablespoon of butter. Bake for about 25 minutes, until the fish flakes when pressed with a fork. Squeeze lemon juice from the lemon wedges over the fish, and serve immediately.

Year-Round Barbecued Brisket

Prep time: 20 minutes

Cooking time: 10 hours

Servings: 4

Nutrients per serving:

Carbohydrates – 3.6 g

Net Carbs – 2.6 g

Fat – 12.3 g

Protein – 35.1 g

Calories – 270

Ingredients:

- 1 (6-ounce) can tomato paste
- ⅓ cup apple cider vinegar
- 1 Tbsp chili powder
- 2 tsp onion powder
- 2 tsp garlic salt
- 1 tsp freshly ground black pepper
- 1 tsp smoked paprika
- 1 tsp cayenne pepper
- 2 Tbsp stevia
- 2 Tbsp whole grain soy flour
- 1 (5-pound) beef brisket

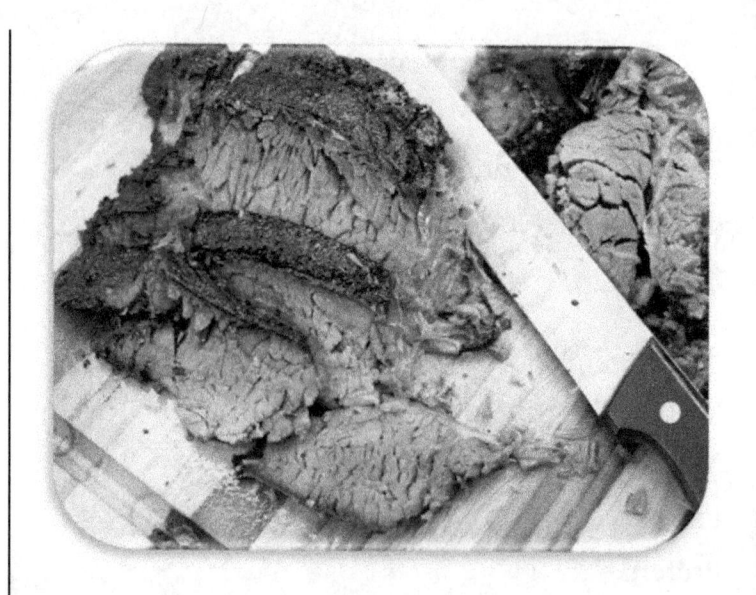

Instructions:

1. Place the tomato paste, vinegar, chili powder, onion powder, garlic salt, black pepper, paprika, cayenne pepper, stevia, and flour in a slow cooker. Whisk to combine. Remove ¼ cup of the sauce to pour over the brisket.
2. Add the brisket, and top with the removed sauce. Set the slow cooker to low, and cook 9 to 10 hours, until the meat is very tender. Shred or slice and serve immediately.

Salmon with Rosemary

Prep time: 15 minutes

Cooking time: 20 minutes

Servings: 2

Nutrients per serving:

Carbohydrates – 1 g

Net Carbs – 0.7 g

Fat – 7.2 g

Protein – 23.3 g

Calories – 227

Ingredients:

- ¼ tsp salt
- 2 tsp rosemary
- 2 tsp lemon juice
- 2 tsp olive oil
- 2 Tbsp minced garlic
- ½ pound salmon fillet
- 1 small pinch pepper

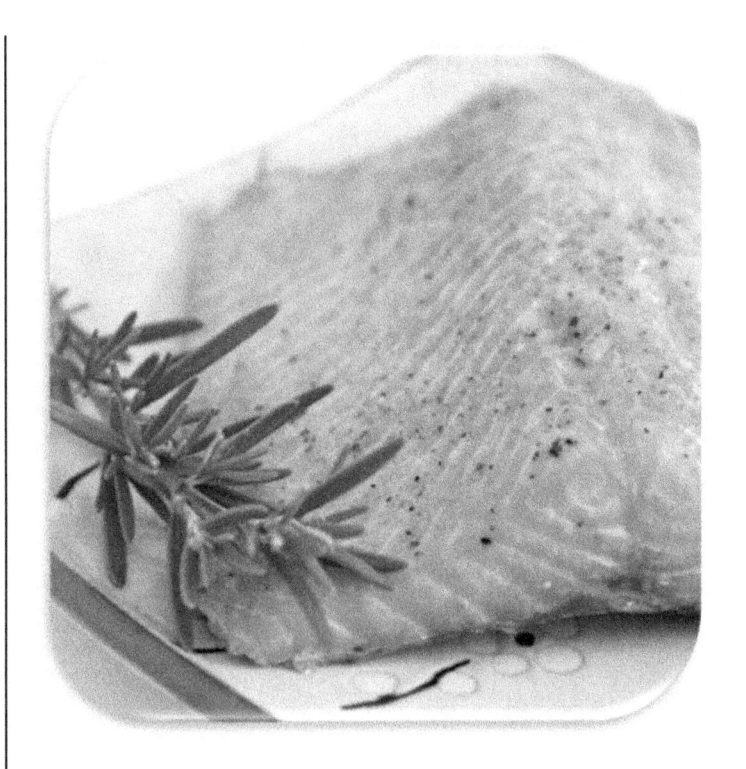

Instructions:

1. Cut salmon in half.
2. In a bowl, combine the rosemary, lemon juice, olive oil, salt, garlic and pepper.
3. Use a brush to apply the mixture into the salmon.
4. Place the fillets on a broiler pan and bake in the ove at 350° F for 20 minutes. Serve.

DESSERTS

Chocolate Chip Cookies

Prep time: 25 minutes

Cooking time: 12 minutes

Servings: 24

Nutrients per serving:

Carbohydrates – 2.5 g

Net Carbs – 1.4 g

Fat – 10.1 g

Protein – 2.4 g

Calories – 111

Ingredients:

- Olive oil spray
- ½ cup coconut oil, at room temperature
- 2 large eggs
- 1 tsp vanilla extract
- ½ tsp almond extract (optional)
- 1½ cups almond flour
- ¼ cup stevia
- ½ tsp baking soda
- 1 tsp ground cinnamon
- ¼ tsp salt
- ½ cup sugar-free chocolate chips

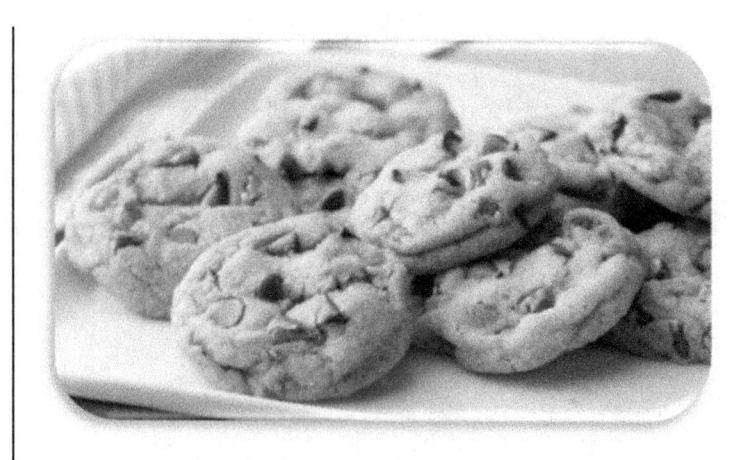

Instructions:

1. Preheat the oven to 375°F. Coat a baking sheet with olive oil spray. Place next four ingredients in a bowl, and beat with a hand mixer for about 1 minute.
2. Mix together the remaining ingredients (except chocolate chips). Beat the almond flour mixture into the wet ingredients until the dough comes together.
3. Drop the cookie dough onto the prepared baking sheet by teaspoonfuls, Gently flatten the cookies by pressing with a fork or spatula. Top each cookie with chocolate chips. Bake 10 minutes, until lightly browned. Let cool completely before serving.

Chocolate-Orange Soufflés

Prep time: 20 minutes

Cooking time: 13 minutes

Servings: 6

Nutrients per serving:

Carbohydrates – 11 g

Net Carbs – 3 g

Fat – 18 g

Protein – 5 g

Calories – 210

Ingredients:

- 5 Tbsp butter, plus more for ramekins
- ⅓ cup granular sugar substitute, plus more for ramekins
- 6½ ounces low-carb or sugar-free chocolate bars
- 1 tsp orange extract
- 5 large eggs, separated
- ¼ tsp cream of tartar

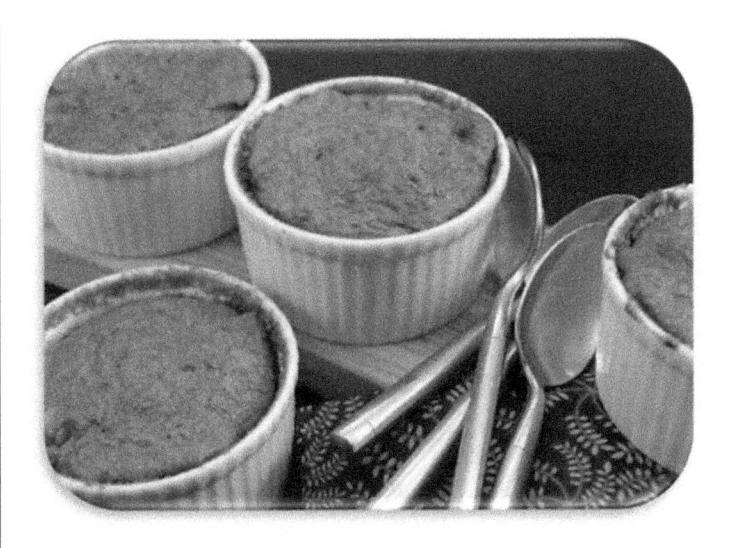

Instructions:

1. Heat oven to 425°F. Lightly butter 6 ramekins; coat the insides with sugar substitute. Set on a baking sheet.
2. Melt chocolate, butter, and orange extract in a small saucepan over low heat. Transfer to a medium bowl. Whisk in egg yolks; set aside.
3. Add egg whites and cream of tartar into another medium bowl; whip with an electric mixer on high speed until frothy. Slowly add sugar substitute; whip until soft peaks form, about 3 minutes. Add one-third of the egg whites into chocolate mixture; gently fold in remaining whites. Divide batter among ramekins; bake until puffed and set, about 13 minutes. Serve right away.

Lickety-Split Vanilla Ice Cream

Prep time: 20 minutes

Cooking time: none

Servings: 8

Nutrients per serving:

Carbohydrates – 4 g

Net Carbs – 4 g

Fat – 36 g

Protein – 2 g

Calories – 340

Ingredients:

- 3¼ cups heavy cream
- ½ cup plus 1 Tbsp granular sugar substitute
- Pinch salt
- ½ tsp pure vanilla extract

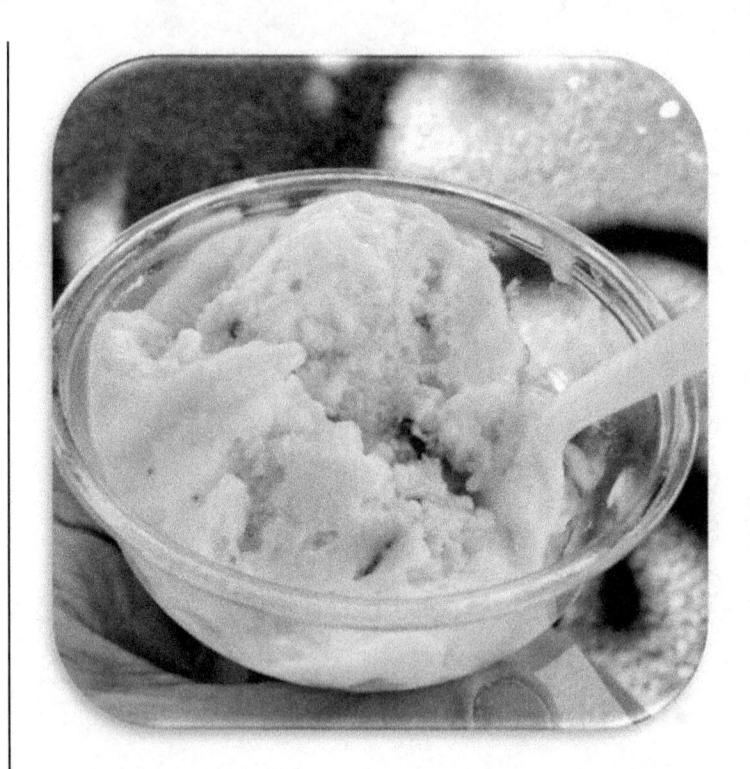

Instructions:

1. Combine cream, sugar substitute, salt, and vanilla in a medium bowl and refrigerate until very well chilled, at least 1 hour.
2. Process according to the instructions for your ice cream maker.
3. Transfer to a container and freeze until ready to serve. Scoop into dessert dishes.

Cranberry-Orange Fool

Prep time: 20 minutes

Cooking time: 10 minutes

Servings: 4

Nutrients per serving:

Carbohydrates – 5 g

Net Carbs – 4 g

Fat – 22 g

Protein – 1 g

Calories – 220

Ingredients:

- 1 cup fresh or frozen cranberries
- ⅓ cup water
- 2 tsp freshly grated orange zest
- 1 cup heavy cream, chilled
- 2 Tbsp granular sugar substitute
- ½ tsp pure vanilla extract

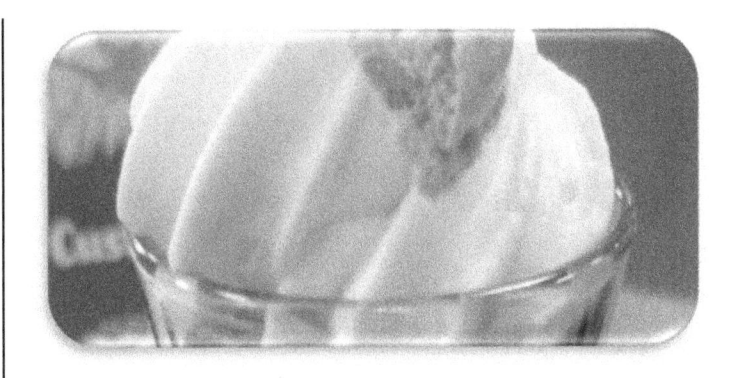

Instructions:

1. Simmer cranberries and water over medium-high heat until mixture thickens and cranberries pop, 5–10 minutes. Transfer to a food processor or blender and purée. Pour into a medium bowl. Add orange zest and stir to blend.
2. Meanwhile, whip cream, sugar substitute, and vanilla with an electric mixer on medium-high speed until soft peaks form.
3. Fold one-third of the whipped cream into cranberries; fold in remaining cream. Scoop into dessert bowls and serve, or refrigerate for up to 4 hours.

Mini-Muffin-Tin Chocolate Brownies

Prep time: 20 minutes

Cooking time: 10 minutes

Servings: 8

Nutrients per serving:

Carbohydrates – 17 g

Net Carbs – 2 g

Fat – 17 g

Protein – 4 g

Calories – 190

Ingredients:

- 4 Tbsp (½ stick) butter, plus more for muffin tin
- 8½ ounces sugar-free or low-carb dark chocolate
- 3 large eggs
- ⅛ tsp salt
- 1 Tbsp flour

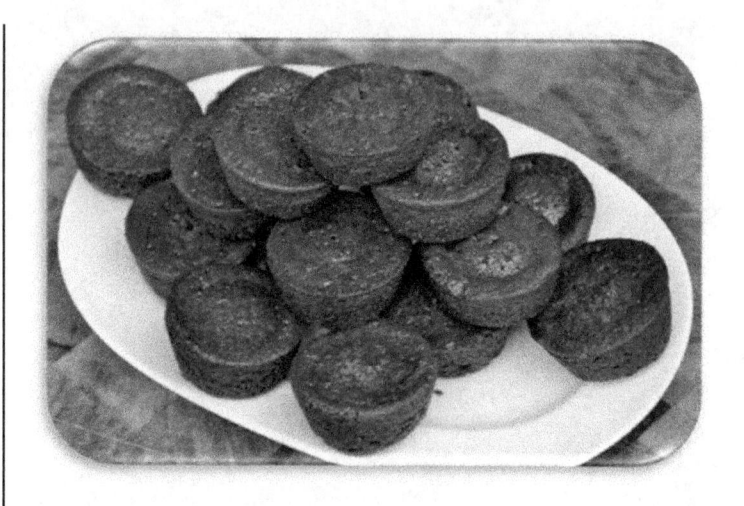

Instructions:

1. Heat oven to 375°F. Lightly butter two 12-cup mini-muffin tins; set aside.
2. Melt butter and chocolate over low heat; let cool slightly.
3. Beat eggs and salt with an electric mixer on high speed. Add flour; beat on low speed just to combine. Add cooled chocolate; whisk on low speed to combine.
4. Divide batter among muffin cups (it will not fill them). Bake until tops are puffed and cracked, about 8–10 minutes. Cool in tin for 5 minutes; transfer to a wire rack to cool completely, about 20 minutes. Serve.

Vanilla Meringues

Prep time: 20 minutes

Cooking time: 1 hour

Servings: 24

Nutrients per serving:

Carbohydrates – 1 g

Net Carbs – 1 g

Fat – 0 g

Protein – 1 g

Calories – 10

Ingredients:

- 3 large egg whites
- 1-½ tsp clear or regular vanilla extract
- ¼ tsp cream of tartar
- Salt, to taste
- ⅔ cup sugar substitute

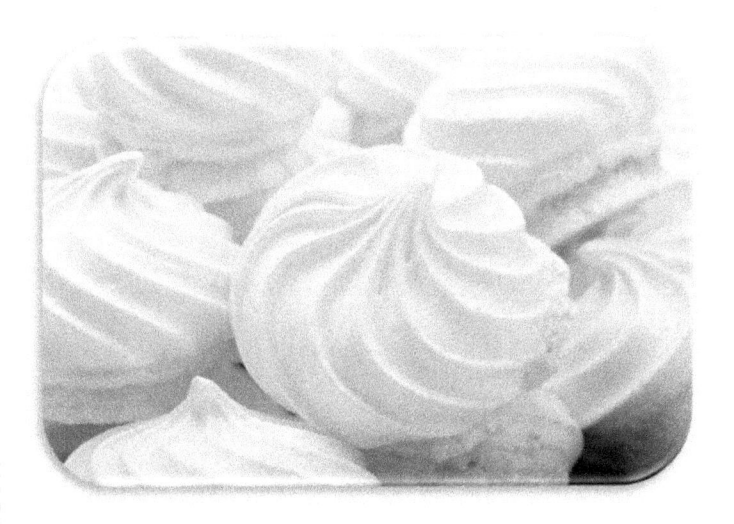

Instructions:

1. Heat oven to 200°F. Line two baking sheets with parchment paper; set aside.
2. Combine egg whites, sugar substitute, vanilla and salt in a large bowl; beat with an electric mixer until medium peaks form. Dollop generous tablespoonfuls of meringue onto baking sheets; bake until dry and crisp, about 1 hour. Cool completely on the baking sheet. Serve.

Apple Crumble

Prep time: 20 minutes

Cooking time: 35 minutes

Servings: 24

Nutrients per serving:

Carbohydrates – 11 g

Net Carbs – 7.3 g

Fat – 19.7 g

Protein – 6.2 g

Calories – 227

Ingredients:

Filling

- Olive oil spray
- 1 medium zucchini, peeled and diced
- 1 green apple, cored and diced
- 3 Tbsp stevia
- 1 Tbsp ground cinnamon
- 1 Tbsp wheat bran
- 1 Tbsp coconut oil
- ⅓ cup water
- 1 tsp vanilla extract

Crust

- 1 cup almond flour
- 2 Tbsp stevia
- 2 tsp whole grain soy flour
- ¼ tsp salt
- ¼ cup unsalted butter, chilled, cut into chunks

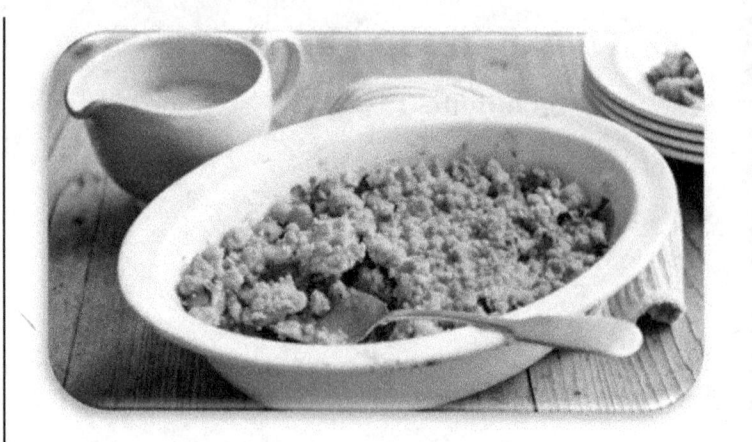

Instructions:

1. Preheat the oven to 350°F. Coat an 8-by-8-inch pan with olive oil spray. Place the zucchini, apple, stevia, cinnamon, and wheat bran in a medium bowl. Mix well.
2. Heat the coconut oil in a skillet over medium heat. Cook the zucchini-apple mixture, tossing well, 1 to 2 minutes. Reduce the heat to low, pour in the water, and cover. Simmer 6 to 8 minutes, until the apple and zucchini are tender and a thick sauce forms. Set aside.
3. Pulse all the crust ingredients in a food processor until a crumbly dough forms. Press half the crust mixture into the prepared pan. Bake 10 to 15 minutes. Spoon the zucchini-apple mixture over the crust, and sprinkle the remaining crust mixture on top. Bake for another 8–10 minutes, until the top starts to brown. Serve immediately.

Double Chocolate Brownies

Prep time: 25 minutes

Cooking time: 25 minutes

Servings: 18

Nutrients per serving:

Carbohydrates – 3.3 g

Net Carbs – 2.1 g

Fat – 10.7 g

Protein – 2.8 g

Calories – 108

Ingredients:

- Olive oil spray
- 4 ounces unsweetened chocolate, chopped
- ½ cup unsalted butter
- ¼ cup canned coconut milk
- ½ cup stevia
- ¼ cup almond flour
- 3 Tbsp unsweetened cocoa powder, divided
- 1 tsp baking powder
- 4 large eggs, whisked

Instructions:

1. Preheat the oven to 325°F. Coat an 8-by-8-inch pan with olive oil spray. Place the chocolate, butter, and coconut milk in a bowl and microwave on high power for approximately 2 minutes. Whisk well, and cool for 5 minutes while you prepare the dry ingredients.

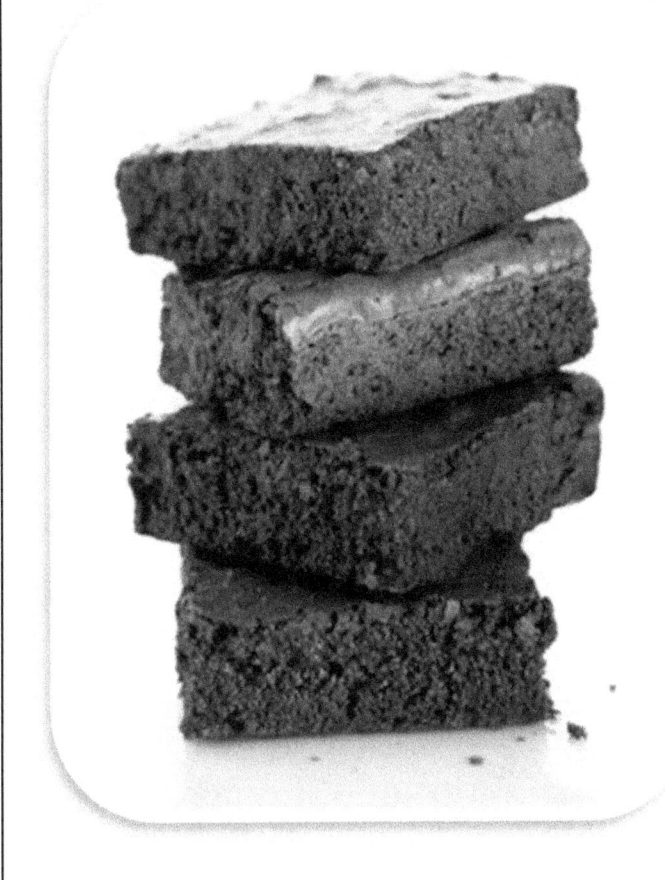

2. Place the stevia, almond flour, 2 tablespoons of the cocoa powder, and baking powder in a large bowl, and mix well. Add in the eggs and the cooled chocolate. Transfer to the prepared pan, and smooth the top with a spatula. Bake for 25 minutes. Let cool, then cut into 18 pieces (three rows of six brownies). Sprinkle with the remaining cocoa powder. Serve.

Salted Caramel Cheesecake Bites

Prep time: 25 minutes
Cooking time: none
Servings: 18

Nutrients per serving:

Carbohydrates – 1.1 g
Net Carbs – 0.9 g
Fat – 7.6 g
Protein – 2.6 g
Calories – 81

Ingredients:

- ½ cup heavy cream
- ⅓ cup plain protein powder
- 2 Tbsp stevia
- 6 ounces full-fat cream cheese, room temperature
- ⅓ cup chopped almonds or macadamia nuts
- 1 Tbsp sugar-free caramel syrup
- 1 tsp vanilla extract
- ⅛ tsp xanthan gum (optional)
- ¼ tsp sea salt or Maldon sea salt flakes

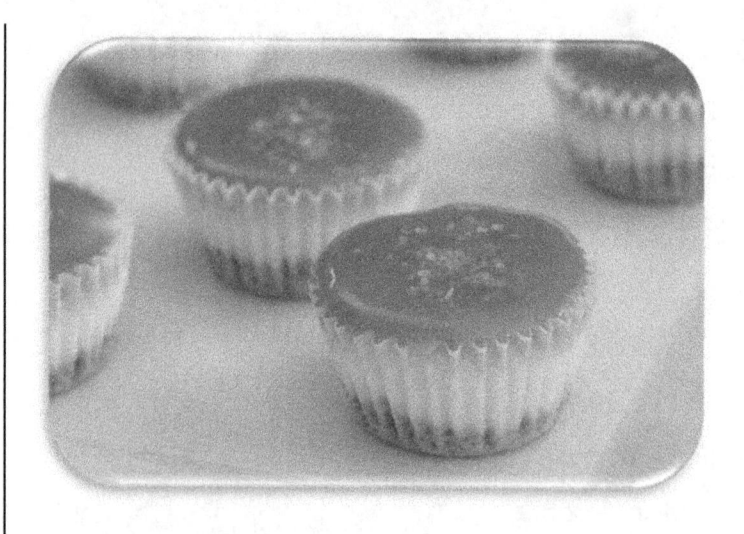

Instructions:

1. Place the heavy cream in a large mixing bowl with the protein powder and stevia. Whisk until smooth. Add the cream cheese, almonds or macadamia nuts, caramel syrup, and vanilla extract, and blend until smooth. Sprinkle the mixture with the xanthan gum, if desired, and mix again for about 30 seconds. The mixture will thicken slightly.
2. Cover a tray that will fit into your freezer with a sheet of wax paper. Use a soup spoon to scoop the mixture onto the tray, make 18 mounds. Alternatively, you can use two silicone candy molds or coat an empty ice cube tray with olive oil spray, and press spoonfuls of the cheesecake mixture into 18 of the molds. Sprinkle with the sea salt. Freeze at least one hour before serving.

Mexican Wedding Cookies

Prep time: 20 minutes

Cooking time: 18 minutes

Servings: 22

Nutrients per serving:

Carbohydrates – 4.2 g

Net Carbs – 2.4 g

Fat – 11.1 g

Protein – 4.4 g

Calories – 124

Ingredients:

- 2 cups almond flour
- 1 cup finely chopped walnuts
- ¼ cup whole grain soy flour
- 1 tsp baking powder
- 1 tsp ground cardamom
- ¼ tsp salt
- ¼ cup unsalted butter, softened
- 1 large egg
- 1 tsp vanilla extract
- ½ cup stevia, divided
- 1 Tbsp ground cinnamon

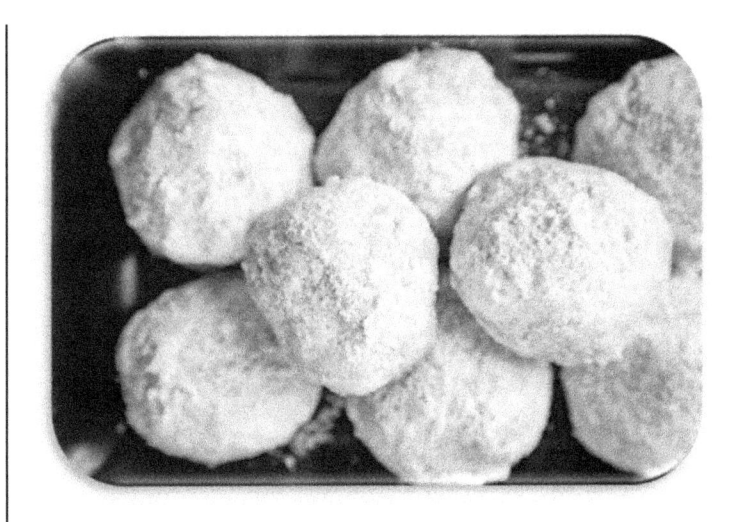

Instructions:

1. Preheat the oven to 325°F, and line two baking sheets with parchment paper.
2. In a bowl, whisk together the almond flour, walnuts, soy flour, baking powder, cardamom, and salt.
3. In another bowl, beat the butter for about 2 minutes. Beat in the egg, vanilla extract, and half the stevia. Then beat in the almond flour mixture until the dough comes together. Form the dough into ¾-inch balls, and place on the baking sheets about 1 inch apart.
4. Bake for about 18 minutes, until just lightly golden brown. In a medium bowl, add the remaining stevia and cinnamon, and mix well. Roll the cookies around in the cinnamon mixture to coat. Transfer to a plate to cool completely. Serve.

CONCLUSION

Thank you for reading this book and having the patience to try the recipes.

I do hope that you have had as much enjoyment reading and experimenting with the meals as I have had writing the book.

If you would like to leave a comment, you can do so at the Order section->Digital orders, in your account.

Stay safe and healthy!

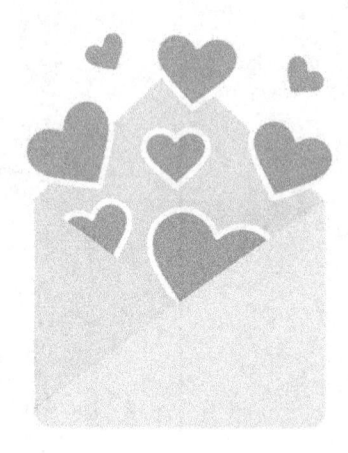

Recipe Index

A

Almond-Crusted Catfish Fingers 67
Apple Crumble 80
Asparagus with Burrata Cheese and Kale Pesto 40
Athenian Salad 51
Atkins Yorkshire Pudding 29

B

Baked Bluefish with Garlic and Lime 68
Baked Salmon with Mustard-Nut Crust 69
Beef Bourguignon 70
Belgian Waffles 19
Birdies in a Basket 30
Braised Lettuce 36
Broiler Huevos Rancheros 25

C

Caprese Salad 52
Cauliflower Bisque 42
Cauliflower Rice Scrambles 24
Cheese Pancake 26
Chicken Vegetable Soup 45
Chicken-Fried Steak 64
Chinese Hot-and-Sour Soup 47
Chocolate Chip Cookies 74
Chocolate-Orange Soufflés 75
Cold Roasted Tomato Soup 50
Cranberry-Orange Fool 77
Cranberry-Orange Loaf 27
Cream of Broccoli Soup 49
Creamy Cheddar Cheese Soup 48
Crunchy Tropical Berry and Almond Breakfast Parfait .. 23
Cucumber-Dill Salad 56

D

Double Chocolate Brownies 81

F

Flaxseed Pancake 20
Fontina-and-Prosciutto-Stuffed Veal Chops 66

J

Jalapeño Cheddar Broccoli Soup 41
Jerk Chicken 62

L

Lickety-Split Vanilla Ice Cream 76

M

Mexican Wedding Cookies 83

Mini-Muffin-Tin Chocolate Brownies 78
Mixed Power Greens Prosciutto-Wrapped Chicken Tenders 59
Mushroom-Herb-Stuffed Chicken Breasts 61

O

Old Bay Shrimp Salad 53

P

Pancakes With Ricotta-Apricot Filling 28
Peanut-Strawberry Breakfast Bars 22

R

Roast Beef with Greek Yogurt- Horseradish Sauce 63
Roasted Cauliflower 37
Roasted Fennel and Cod with Moroccan Olives 71
Roasted Lemon-Garlic Brussels Sprouts 33

S

Salmon with Rosemary 73
Salsa Verde Chicken Soup 44
Salted Caramel Cheesecake Bites 82
Sautéed Baby Bok Choy with Garlic and Lemon Zest 34
Sautéed Greens with Pecans 31
Sautéed Spinach with Caramelized Shallots 38
Shaved Fennel Salad with Lemon Dressing 55
Shishito Peppers with Hot Paprika Mayonnaise 39
Slaw with Vinegar Dressing 57
Slow-Cooked Pork Shoulder 65
Spicy Korean Soup with Scallions 43
Stir-Fried Broccolini with Cashews 32
Swiss Chard with Pine Nuts 35

T

Thai Coconut-Shrimp Soup 46
Tomato and Red Onion Salad 60

V

Vanilla Meringues 79

W

Watercress Bacon Salad with Ranch Dressing 54
Wedge Salad with Gorgonzola Dressing 58
Whole-Wheat Currant Scones 21

Y

Year-Round Barbecued Brisket 72

Conversion Tables

VOLUME EQUIVALENTS (LIQUID)

US STANDARD	US STANDARD (OUNCES)	METRIC
2 tablespoons	1 fl. oz.	30 mL
¼ cup	2 fl. oz.	60 mL
½ cup	4 fl. oz.	120 mL
1 cup	8 fl. oz.	240 mL
1½ cups	12 fl. oz.	355 mL
2 cups or 1 pint	16 fl. oz.	475 mL
4 cups or 1 quart	32 fl. oz.	1 L
1 gallon	128 fl. oz.	4 L

OVEN TEMPERATURES

FAHRENHEIT (°F)	CELSIUS (°C) APPROXIMATE
250 °F	120 °C
300 °F	150 °C
325 °F	165 °C
350 °F	180 °C
375 °F	190 °C
400 °F	200 °C
425 °F	220 °C
450 °F	230 °C

VOLUME EQUIVALENTS (LIQUID)

US STANDARD	METRIC (APPROXIMATE)
1/8 teaspoon	0.5 mL
¼ teaspoon	1 mL
½ teaspoon	2 mL
2/3 teaspoon	4 mL
1 teaspoon	5 mL
1 tablespoon	15 mL
¼ cup	59 mL
1/3 cup	79 mL
½ cup	118 mL
2/3 cup	156 mL
¾ cup	177 mL
1 cup	235 mL
2 cups or 1 pint	475 mL
3 cups	700 mL
4 cups or 1 quart	1 L
½ gallon	2 L
1 gallon	4 L

WEIGHT EQUIVALENTS

US STANDARD	METRIC (APPROXIMATE)
½ ounce	15 g
1 ounce	30 g
2 ounces	60 g
4 ounces	115 g
8 ounces	225 g
12 ounces	340 g
16 ounces or 1 pound	455 g

Other Books by Adele Baker

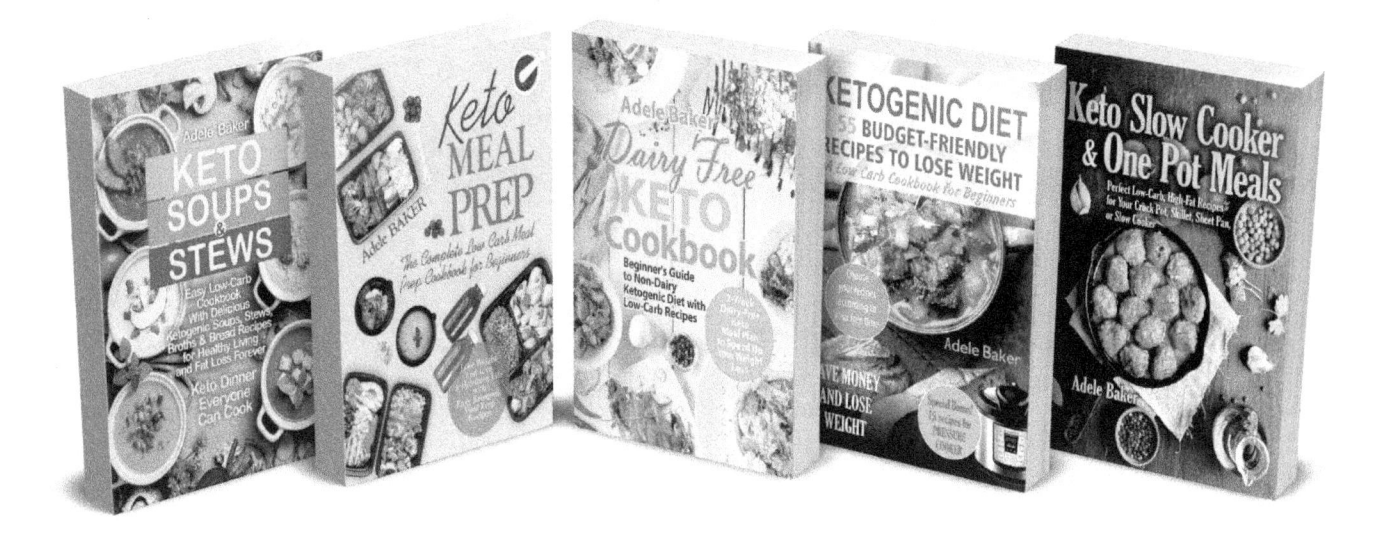

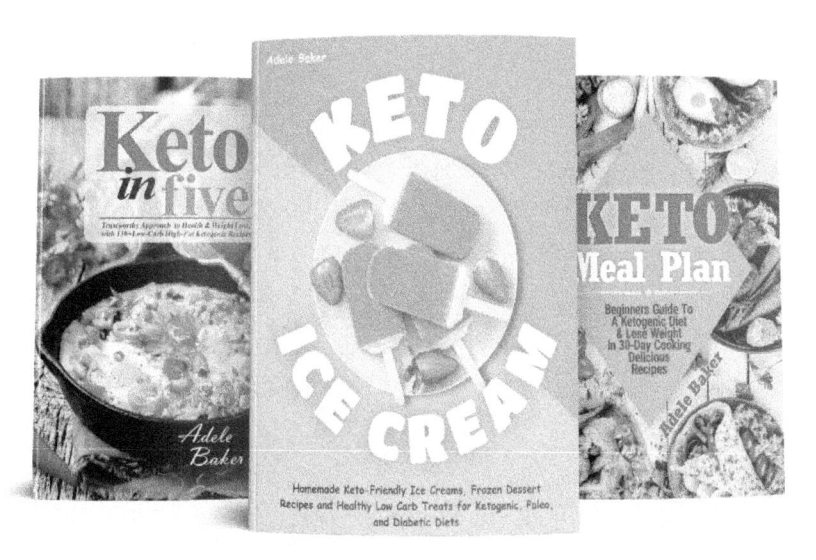

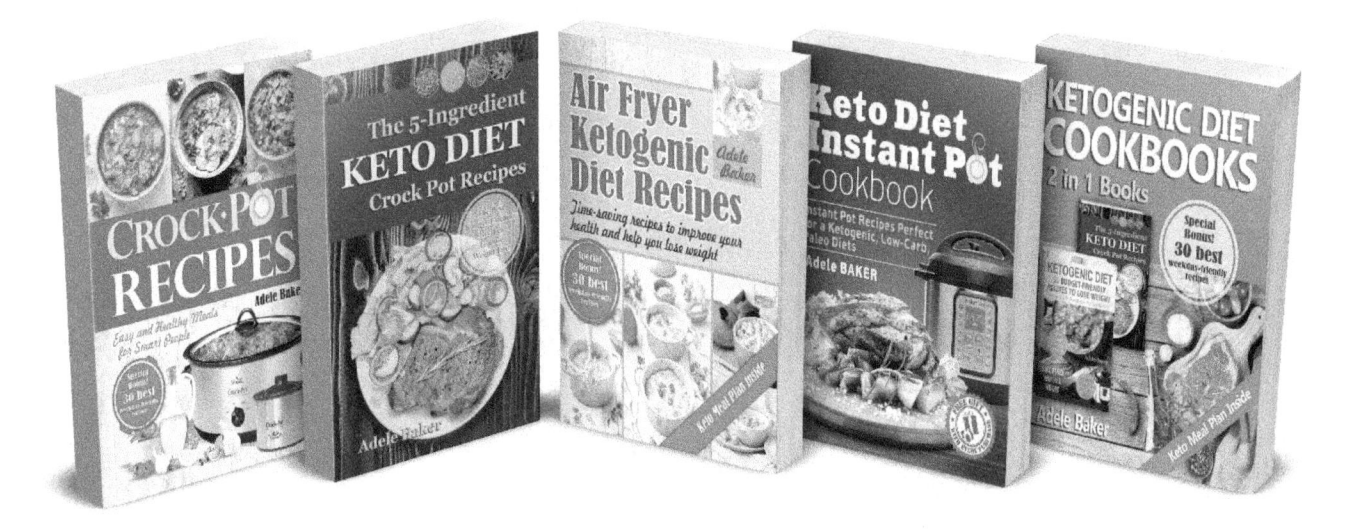

CPSIA information can be obtained
at www.ICGtesting.com
Printed in the USA
BVHW061353081019
560524BV00011B/305/P

9 781087 803029